To
Lesley Seeney my loyal and accommodating secretary who has for many years uncomplainingly undertaken my work.

Preface

Up to the early 1980s neuropsychological assessments of persons with intellectual disability (ID) usually meant an assessment for developmental delay, of intelligence (intelligence quotient testing) or of level of adaptive behavior. Popular tests included the Stanford-Binet, Wechsler Intelligence Scales, Bayley Scales of Infant Development, the Griffin Mental Developmental Scales, and the Vineland Social Maturity Scale. These were assessments of the "overall" level of ability. Arthur Dalton in New York was one of a few pioneering clinicians who at this time, focused on the development of tests for specific areas of cognition in persons with ID. Following his work, subsequent researchers, in the latter part of the twentieth century, have proposed and developed a number of measures not only to detect the level of cognitive abilities but also to measure decline; a perquisite to the diagnosis of dementia.

At the beginning of the twenty-first century as demonstrated in this book, several neuropsychological measures have been developed to aid the clinical diagnosis of dementia/dementia in Alzheimer's disease (AD). Neuropsychological assessments no longer remain the sole responsibility of psychologists, as psychiatrists, researchers, ID nurses, neuroscientists, all now play a part in the development and administration of specific tests.

As a consequence of the development in neuropsychological tests of older persons with ID, there has been a steady growth in the publication of research reports, case studies, reviews, drug trials, using such instruments. It is now standard practice for at least one neuropsychological measure to be used in standard clinical practice, and indeed internationally recognized diagnostic criteria for the diagnosis of dementia in AD often requires that at least one of these measures are used as part of the diagnostic pathway.

It would be an injustice to the researchers and clinicians who developed these tests for their tests to be appraised by myself. This book, therefore, contains a review of the most important neuropsychological measures used in the assessment of dementia by the researchers who developed or who are the principle researchers associated with the tests. It is a tribute to such researchers that they themselves felt the neuropsychological assessments of dementia in persons with ID remains an important area of clinical care and as a result kindly contributed to this book.

The overall organization of this book is that the most popular and most widely used tests have been given precedence in chapter order as compared to the newer,

less well-developed tests. Test researchers were asked to cover a number of important areas but also to discuss their personal views on the test. Where possible, to aid
readers, a sample page of each test has been included in the "Appendix" section.
This gives the readers a chance to catch sight of the layout of at least a few of the
test questions.

A few comments on terminology adopted in this text. The term "Alzheimer's disease" has been used to denote the neuropathological disease process while "Dementia
in Alzheimer's disease" (DAD) has been used to refer to the clinical aspects of the
neurodegenerative condition. Dementia in Alzheimer's type (DAT) is used where it is
specifically used as a diagnostic term in the test measure. It is accepted that such
terms have not as yet gained universal acceptance. Further the term "intellectual
disability(ies)" is used in this text to be synonymous with "mental retardation,"
"learning disabilities," "mental handicap," and "intellectual handicap."

Acknowledgment

I am indebted to the scholarly clinicians and researchers who have contributed so benevolently and whose names are listed at the beginning of this book. Without their support and contribution Neuropsychological Assessments of Down Syndrome and Intellectual Disabilities would not exist.

Contents

Contributors

Sarah L. Ball, DM, FRCP, FRCPath, FRCPCH
Department of Psychiatry, University of Cambridge, Cambridge, UK

Diana B. Burt, BS, MS, PhD
Volunteer Faculty—Department of Psychiatry, University of Texas,
Houston, TX, USA

Mary Cosgrove, MD MSc (Psychotherapy), FRCPI, MRCPsych
Department of Psychiatry, HSE Dublin North-East and Beaumont Hospital,
Dublin, Ireland

Arthur J. Dalton, BSc, BA, MA, PhD
Department of Molecular Biology Department, Center for Aging Studies,
New York State Institute for Basic Research in Developmental Disabilities,
Staten Island, NY, USA

Darlynne A. Devenny, MA, PhD
Department of Psychology, New York State Institute for Basic Research
in Developmental Disabilities, Staten Island, NY, USA

Heleen M. Evenhuis, PhD
Department of Intellectual Disability Medicine, Erasmus University
Medical Center, Rotterdam, the Netherlands

Harry A.L. Eurlings, PhD
Department of Psychology, Hooge Burch Centre for the Intellectually Disabled,
Zwammerdam, Zuid-Holland, the Netherlands

Angela Gedye, PhD, Rpsych
Private Practice Psychologist, Vancouver, British Columbia, Canada

Maria Luisa Hanney, MB BSc, MRCPsych, PhD
Consultant and Senior Lecturer in Old Age Psychiatry for people
with learning disability, King's College London and Northgate Hospital,
Northumberland, UK

Anthony J. Holland, BSc, MBBS, MRCP, MRCPsych, MPhil, DipHumClinGenet,
Department of Psychiatry, University of Cambridge, Cambridge, UK

Emoke Jozsvai, PhD, CPsych
Department of Psychology, Surrey Place Centre, Toronto, Ontario, Canada

Polyxeni Kartakis, PhD
Department of Psychology, Surrey Place Centre, Toronto, Ontario, Canada

Maria M.F. Kengen, PhD
Department of Psychology, The Bridges Care Centre, Nieuwveen,
Zuid-Holland, the Netherlands

Sharon J. Krinsky-McHale, PhD
Department of Psychology, New York State Institute for
Basic Research in Developmental Disabilities, Staten Island, NY, USA

Philip McCallion, PhD, MSW
Center for Excellence in Aging Services, University at Albany,
New York, NY, USA

Mary McCarron, PhD, BNS, RNID, RGN
School of Nursing and Midwifery Studies, Trinity College, Dublin, Ireland

Peter B. Moore, MB, BS, BSc, PhD, FRCPsych
Department of Psychiatry, Northumbria University, Newcastle-upon-Tyne, UK

Niamh M. Mulryan, MRCPsych, MB, BCh, BAO, MA, MSc
Department of Psychiatry, Daughters of Charity Services,
St Vincent's Centre, Dublin, Ireland

Vee P. Prasher
Liverpool John Moore University, C/o The Greenfields,
Monyhull, Kings Norton, Birmingham, UK

Evelyn M. Reilly, PG.DIP, RNID
St. Joseph's Centre, Daughters of Charity Service, Clonsilla, Dublin, Ireland

Nicole Schupf, PhD, MPH, DrPH
Department of Clinical Epidemiology, Taub Institute for research on
Alzheimer's disease and the Aging Brain, Columbia University
Medical Centre, New York, NY, USA

Wayne Silverman, PhD
Department of Psychology and Intellectual Disabilities Research,
Kennedy Krieger Institute, Baltimore, MD, USA

Janette F. Tyrrell, MD, MRCPI, BaMOD, MRCPsych
Department of Psychiatry, St Michael's House, Dublin, Ireland

Stephen P. Tyrer, MB, BChir., DPM, LMCC, FRCPsych
Department of Psychiatry, Northumbria University, Newcastle-upon-Tyne, UK

Tina K. Urv, PhD
Department of Psychiatry, University of Massachusetts Medical School-EK
Shriver Center, Waltham, MA, USA

Warren B. Zigman, BA, MA, MPhil, PhD
Department of Psychology, New York State Institute for Basic Research
in Developmental Disabilities, Staten Island, NY, USA

Abbreviations

ABDQ   Adaptive Behavior Dementia Questionnaire
AD   Alzheimer's disease
ABS   Adaptive Behavior Scale

CAMDEX-DS   Cambridge Examination for Mental Disorders of Older People
              with Down's Syndrome and Others with Intellectual Disabilities

DAD   Dementia in Alzheimer's disease
DAT   Dementia of Alzheimer's type
DMR   Dementia Questionnaire for Mentally Retarded Persons
DS   Down syndrome
DSDS   Down Syndrome Dementia Scale
DSM-IV   Diagnostic and Statistical Manual of Mental Disorders—Fourth
              Edition

ICD-10   International Classification of Diseases and Related Health
              Problems—Tenth Revision

ID   Intellectual disabilities
IQ   Intelligence quotient

MCI   Mild Cognitive Impairment
MMSE   Mini-Mental State Examination

SIB   Severe Impairment Battery

TSI   Test for Severe Impairment

Chapter 1
Overview of the Neuropsychological Assessment of Dementia in Intellectual Disability

M.L. Hanney, S.P. Tyrer, and P.B. Moore

Introduction

Dementia is a difficult diagnosis to make in someone with reduced intellectual capacity. There is no definition of dementia that is specific for individuals with intellectual disabilities (ID). In 1997, a working group under the auspices of the Scientific Study of Intellectual Disability and the American Association on Mental Retardation addressed the problem of lack of standardized criteria for the diagnosis of dementia in individuals with ID. This working group proposed the use of the *International Classification of Diseases*, 10th edition (ICD-10) criteria[1] for this purpose as opposed to *Diagnostic and Statistical Manual of Mental Disorders*, 4th edition (DSM-IV) criteria,[2] because ICD-10 criteria[1] places more emphasis on "noncognitive" aspects of dementia (e.g., emotional liability, irritability, and apathy) and uses a two-step diagnostic process. This procedure involves establishing a diagnosis of dementia and then differentiating dementia in Alzheimer's disease (DAD) from other forms of dementia.[3] As such, the process should include a direct assessment of cognitive and noncognitive functioning (level of independent functioning and presence of aberrant behavior). Care must be taken not only in carrying out appropriate tests but also in the interpretation of all results obtained from these. Hence, a specific and detailed knowledge of the differential diagnosis, symptoms, and course of dementia is required of a clinician to interpret clinical findings and results particularly if the actual tests performed have been carried out by nonspecialized workers.[4]

According to the ICD-10 diagnostic guidelines,[1] dementia is a disease of the brain, usually of a chronic or progressive nature, in which there is disturbance of multiple higher cortical functions, including memory, thinking, orientation, comprehension, calculation, learning capacity, language, and judgment. Consciousness is not clouded. Impairments of cognitive function in dementia are commonly accompanied, and occasionally preceded, by deterioration in emotional control, social behavior, or motivation. In assessing the presence or absence of a dementia, special care needs be taken to avoid false-positive identification because of motivational or emotional factors, particularly depression. Furthermore, motor slowness and general physical frailty, rather than loss of intellectual capacity, may account for any deterioration noted in performance.

V.P. Prasher (ed.), *Neuropsychological Assessments of Dementia in Down Syndrome and Intellectual Disabilities*, DOI: 10.1007/978-1-84800-249-4_1, © Springer Science+Business Media, LLC 2009

Typically, the primary requirement for the diagnosis of dementia is evidence of a decline in both memory and thinking which is sufficient to impair personal activities of daily living, such as washing, dressing, eating, personal hygiene, and excretory activities. The impairment of memory usually affects the registration, storage, and retrieval of new information, but previously learned and familiar material may also be lost, particularly in the later stages. Dementia is more than dysmnesia: there is also impairment of thinking and of reasoning capacity, and a reduction in the flow of ideas. The processing of incoming information is impaired, in that the individual finds it increasingly difficult to attend to more than one stimulus at a time, such as taking part in a conversation with several persons, and to shift the focus of attention from one topic to another. Decline in emotional control or motivation, or a change in social behavior, is also required for a diagnosis of dementia. These changes should be manifest in at least one of the following areas:

1. Emotional lability
2. Irritability
3. Apathy and
4. Coarsening of social behavior

The above symptoms and impairments should have been evident for at least 6 months in order to make a confident clinical diagnosis.

When diagnosing dementia in adults with ID, the most important fact to recognize is that the diagnosis requires a change in status. Longitudinal assessments that document both baseline and present cognitive functioning as well as behavioral functioning over a period of at least 6 months is necessary before sufficient information can be obtained to make a confident diagnosis of dementia.[5] This population has varying baseline profiles of abilities and disabilities and varying sensory impairment.[6,7] In addition, they have a wide range of behavioral problems that are atypical, and assessing the clinical significance of such behavior requires a comparison with adulthood functioning in this population.[6]

The perception of cognitive decline in this population will also depend upon the premorbid level of intellectual functioning.[6] Decline in cognitive function and behavior in individuals with mild ID who develop dementia can be very similar to that seen in those of the general population who have the same illness, whereas decline in individuals with more severe ID can present with a very different picture. In order to be meaningful, changes in performance on cognitive testing must be accompanied by changes in everyday independent functioning. To be indicative of dementia, any changes over time must also be greater than those related to normal aging in adults with ID.[6,8]

Our ability to detect dementia in people in the ID population is not only hampered by developmental differences within the group but also by the poor sensitivity and specificity of existing test tools. There is a need for simple and reliable screening instruments for dementia in the ID population that can also be used to follow up their progress, particularly if subjects are being treated with antidementia drugs.

The question whether a screening instrument can be developed to detect dementia among all categories of the ID population is open to debate. Given the heterogeneity of skills, variable preexisting level of independence, the difficulty in establishing cutoff scores and the possible variable clinical early presentation of dementia in this population, it is difficult to imagine that a screening questionnaire could be designed to be applicable to the wide range of individuals with ID.

Two types of tests are used to help with the diagnosis of dementia in people within this group: (1) those administered to informants, and (2) those that rely on direct assessment of the individual. Among these, some tests are used in the general population with or without modification for the use in the ID population and some are developed specifically to be used exclusively within this population.

There are two main types of instruments used for diagnosing dementia in people with ID. One group consists of tools aimed to give a global assessment of cognitive performance, whereas the other comprise tests that specifically assess certain cognitive functions known to deteriorate earlier in dementia, such as recent memory, attention, or executive function. In the same way some questionnaires that assess global independent level of functioning are used as benchmarks for future comparison as opposed to those that assess abilities that may decline early in the disease. Applicability of test material that is already available and standardized in the general population is an important consideration but the transferability of norms from this source to persons with ID is open to debate.[4]

Thompson[9] published an extensive review of the most commonly used instruments to diagnose dementia in the ID population. One of the most frequently employed informant-rated screening tools specifically developed for people with ID is the Dementia Questionnaire for Mentally Retarded Persons recently termed the Dementia Questionnaire for People with Intellectual Disabilities (DMR; Chapter 3).[10] However, sensitivity in single assessments is variable and cutoff scores need further optimization. In persons with Down syndrome (DS), the Dementia Scale for Down Syndrome (DSDS; Chapter 4)[7] has good specificity but mediocre sensitivity. The Test for Severe Impairment (TSI; Chapter 8)[11] and Severe Impairment Battery (SIB)[12] are two direct assessment tools that show promise as screening instruments, but need further evaluation.[13] Other direct instruments borrowed from the general population include the Cambridge Cognitive Examination (CAMCOG),[14] the Rivermead Behavioral Memory Test,[15,16] Wechsler Adult Intelligence Scale-Revised (WAIS-R),[17] Raven Colored Progressive Matrices (RCPM),[18] Middlesex Elderly Assessment of Mental State (MEAMS),[19] and Hampshire Social Services Assessment.[20]

Because of difficulties regarding cognitive assessment in people with ID, alternative methods of diagnosing and monitoring the progression of dementia in this population have been proposed.[21] These include assessing changes in emotional functioning[22] and adaptive behavior.[23] Caregiver assessment of patients' overall level of functioning can also be measured by using instruments such as the DSDS,[7] The Early Signs of Dementia Checklist (ESDC),[24] and the DMR questionnaire.[25] The standardized administration of a mental status instrument is preferable to a less formal assessment of cognitive ability because it allows confident comparisons of results over time.[3]

In their review of instruments for assessing memory problems, Zelinski and Gilewski[26] noted that people who are poorly educated or who have below normal intelligence quotient (IQ) assessments perform poorly on test of mental status and often are likely to be described as cognitively declined when in fact they are not.[27] These authors proposed that the evaluation of dementia in people with ID requires use of a carer interview as well as direct assessment. Carers can report on cognitive decline independently of premorbid intelligence ability.

The DSDS[7] and the DMR[10] are the best known carer assessment instruments. These two instruments, together with the Modified Cambridge Cognitive Examination for Mental Disorders of the Elderly,[28,29] are recommended tools to assess severity of dementia in people with ID in the Report by National Institute for Health and Clinical Excellence-Social Care Institute for Excellence published in 2006.[30]

Certain neuropsychological tests that were originally devised for the use in the general population have been adapted for the use in people with ID. Examples of such apart from the named above include, the Fuld Object-Memory Evaluation (Modified),[31] the Boston Naming Test (Modified),[32] the McCarthy Verbal Fluency Test,[33] the Simple Commands,[34] and the Purdue Pegboard (Modified).[35] Scales for the assessment of Activities of Daily Living such as the Adaptive Behavior Scale (ABS; Chapter 6)[36] have also been used by some to diagnose dementia in adults with DS.[37,38] Although researchers have shown a decline on the ABS score among their cohort of adults with DS in longitudinal studies, no validated cutoff score according to the ABS is available yet to make a diagnosis of dementia in people with ID. By using neuropsychological tests in a longitudinal study, Devenny and colleagues[39] showed the effect of normal aging in a group of adults with DS.

Psychological Tools

Commonly Used Instruments Administered to Informants

Caregivers, family members, or professionals are important sources of information who can comment on an individual's past performance, abilities and observed changes in everyday functioning. Although informant-based measures should be used cautiously within a retrospective assessment approach, they are useful when repeated over time. However, as baseline measures may not be available when an individual first presents with changes that might indicate dementia, this has led to a heavy reliance on informant-based measures.

As well as the above-mentioned instruments based on information reported by an informant, other instruments include the ESDC[40] and the Multidimensional Observation Scale for Elderly Subjects (MOSES) adapted for adults with DS.[41] These scales incorporate changes in cognitive as well as daily living skills in people with ID. Of these scales, the ESDC[40] has only been used in institutionalized adults with DS, whereas the other three scales have been used in community-based adults with DS. The MOSES[41] is designed for longitudinal use only and has no cutoff score for the diagnosis of dementia.

Dementia Questionnaire for People with Intellectual Disabilities (DMR)

The DMR was developed by Evenhuis[42] as an aid to the diagnosis of dementia in people with ID. This is an English translation of the original test published in Dutch in 1990.[10] The 50 items are grouped in eight subscales divided in two subcategories: (1) cognitive scores: short-term memory; long-term memory; spatial and temporal orientation; and (2) social scores: speech; practical skills; mood; activity and interest; behavior and disturbance. A family member or staffs who knows the patient well scores his or her behavior over the previous 2 months according to a three response categories: 0 points, no deficit; 1 point, moderate deficit; and 2 points, severe deficit. The questionnaire does not require previous training but includes simple instructions. It takes 15–20 min to complete.

The DMR has been evaluated in a number of studies.[25,43,44] Interrater reliability, internal consistency of items, relationship between intellectual level and scores, influence of some physical handicaps on the scores, relationship between diagnosis of dementia and scores, and the relationship between the diagnosis of dementia and scores was investigated in two cross-sectional studies among older residents of three Dutch institutions.[25,45]

This test was specifically designed for use with people with ID and when used together with standardized tools, it has been useful in providing important information for clinicians assessing dementia in people with ID. The test, however, has some drawbacks. Furthermore, the instrument is less sensitive for assessing individuals with dementia in the severe and profound ranges of ID who may never have been able to perform many of the skills assessed in the questionnaire.[44] Thompson[46] and Evenhuis[25] have also pointed out that it is difficult to discern sensitivity of the DMR when used with depressed individuals and they recommend the use of additional tools. Although the author reported results for single cross-sectional scores, Evenhuis[44] recommended that score changes over time should be the most valid criterion, as single assessment cutoff scores could be inaccurate.[13,47] Cutoff scores for dementia should be used cautiously and in conjunction with information gathered from other neuropsychological instruments.[44,48]

Dementia Scale for Down Syndrome

This scale is an informant scored questionnaire that was designed to detect cognitive decline, especially at lower ranges of functioning. The DSDS items were developed for adults with DS mostly with severe or profound ID. In the original validation study 90% of the participants had severe or profound learning disability.[7] Despite its name, the DSDS was not intended solely for use in people with DS. Informants are asked to rate subjects on up to 60 items, 20 of which may indicate early stages of dementia, 20 middle stages, and 20 late stages of dementia. In addition, informants are asked to report whether behaviors are typical of the individual during earlier adulthood, whether these behaviors are currently present or absent, and whether or not the date of onset for the behaviors is known.[49] The scale also includes questions that allow the differentiation between dementia, depression, hearing and vision loss, problems with pain, medication-induced cognitive decline and hypothyroidism.[7] Although the manual requires a chartered psychologist to gather information on changes in behavior from two informants, it has been used in clinical practice and in screening by other mental health professionals.[48,50]

The DSDS appears to be a good screening tool for dementia in people with ID. The advantage of the DSDS is that it does not depend on direct subject participation, which is difficult to achieve for many adults with DS. Also, this scale only takes into account new behaviors that have appeared recently and have lasted for at least 6 months. By using this criteria, the impairments in cognitive and daily living skills which have been present before the index illness can be excluded to avoid a floor effect. It appears that repeated assessments using the DSDS can improve accuracy of diagnosis when compared to a single assessment when the dementia process has progressed further. A high correlation between the diagnosis of DAD and the DSDS findings has been reported in subjects in the middle or late stages of dementia. Disparity in diagnosis has been found between DSDS and the clinical diagnosis when subjects with mild or moderate ID have presented with symptoms of early-stage dementia.

Early Signs of Dementia Checklist

The ESDC[40] is a list of 37 questions with binary scores. It is a checklist that scores clinical signs of mental deterioration and was found to have very good internal consistency and interrater reliability.[40] There appears to be a more comprehensive version consisting of 64 questions, which was used by Hoekman and Maaskant[51] in a current validity and sensitivity study. They found poor agreement with other instruments, but reasonable sensitivity and specificity when compared with expert opinion. Strydom and Hassiotis[13] pointed out the methodological problems of the study such as using a consensus diagnosis of dementia rather than a clinical assessment of mental state and cognition, a small number of participants with dementia and the exclusion of those with severe dementia.

The Short Informant Questionnaire on Cognitive Decline in the Elderly

The Short Informant Questionnaire on Cognitive Decline in the Elderly (IQCODE)[52] has been evaluated by Schultz and colleagues[53] for use in people with ID. In this population, they found mediocre test–retest reliability and poor correlation with current mental status.[54] This is usually measured by informant report and a number of instruments are available. However, none has been adapted for people with ID to screen for dementia.

Comments on Instruments Administered to Informants

Informant-based instruments are often used to complement assessments in the general elderly population, but it is even more important in the assessment of persons with ID. The issue of interrater reliability combined with the change in informant over time may lead to the collection of data that are of poor quality. Both the DSDS and DMR have been thoroughly evaluated. The DMR is the only instrument that has been used in adults with DS and non-DS ID persons. However, as with all single assessments, the sensitivity is variable, and clinical assessment to exclude other causes of decline is essential.

Commonly Used Instruments Administered to ID Persons

A clinical diagnosis of dementia requires evidence of progressive deterioration in a person's cognitive abilities and daily living skills.[1] The most significant problem for the assessment of specific neuropsychological deficits associated with dementia is the variability of intellectual ability and the problems of administering neuropsychological tests to those with severe or profound ID who may not understand verbal commands.[3,55] Poor performance on neuropsychological tests that might indicate dementia might easily be attributable to ID. This is obviously due to the fact that in the case of a person with ID, the mere presence of cognitive impairment does not equate to a diagnosis of dementia because often the impairments have been present throughout the person's life.[48] Sequential testing has been recommended in order to identify decline due to dementia in individuals with ID through the identification of deterioration in scores from a previous baseline using standardized neuropsychological tests.[3] Instruments employed for assessing dementia in the general population such as the Mini-Mental State Examination (MMSE)[56] have proved to be unsuitable for diagnosing dementia in the ID population.[48,57] Because the limitations of the MMSE and other short screening instruments in people with ID, researchers have been investigating and developing alternatives.

The Down Syndrome Mental Status Examination (DSMSE)

This is a neuropsychological test battery developed by Haxby[34] that is used to measure recall for personal information, orientation to season and day of week, short-term memory, language, visuospatial construction, and praxis. It is easy to administer[58] but persons with severe ID frequently score zero.[59]

The Test for Severe Impairment

The TSI was designed by Albert and Cohen in 1992 to assess people with severe dementia in the general population whose MMSE[56] score is less than 10 out of 30.[11] The test takes approximately 10 min and the level of difficulty of the TSI is such that most persons with moderate to severe ID should be able to make a measurable score unless they are in an advance stage of dementia. This instrument contains six sections (Motor Performance, Language Production, Language Comprehension,

Memory, Conceptualization, and General Knowledge) each of which has four items. Only 8 out of the 24 points available required the person to answer a question verbally. This may be of benefit when testing persons with DS whose verbal abilities tend to be relatively poorly developed.

Although designed for the general population with severe dementia the TSI appears to be able to provide a good range of values with almost no floor effect in people with DS. Clear differences are found in those with dementia, those with moderate ID and those with severe ID without dementia. The test has also satisfactory construct validity and reliability in this population. Specifically, in the group with severe ID, the TSI appears to be a good instrument to monitor the progression of dementia longitudinally. However, the properties of the items most consistently answered correctly may signal limitations of the usefulness of the TSI for this subgroup because it is likely that correct answer to these items will not be lost until late in the dementing process. This instrument has particular value in the assessment of dementia in those with severe degrees of ID.

Severe Impairment Battery

The SIB[12] was developed to assess a range of cognitive functioning in patients in the general population with severe dementia who are unable to complete standard neuropsychological tests. There have been three versions of the test and a recently published short version. The test has been translated and validated in Korean, Italian, Spanish, and French populations.[60–62] It relies on direct assessment of the individual and takes into account the specific behavioral and cognitive deficits associated with severe dementia, allowing for nonverbal or partially correct response such as matching. It is brief, taking approximately 30 min to administer (15 min for the short version). It is composed of simple one-step commands which are presented in conjunction with gestured commands. The SIB is divided into six subscales: attention, orientation, language, memory, visuospatial ability, and construction. There are also brief evaluations of praxis and the patients to respond appropriately when his/her name is called (orientation to name).

The psychometric properties of this scale have been assessed in people with DS with and without dementia.[63,64] Witts and Elders[65] concluded that the SIB had good test–retest reliability and criterion validity and that in general terms it is suitable for the neuropsychological cognitive assessment of adults with DS. McKenzie and colleagues[63] in their study concluded that the orientation domain of the SIB may be a discriminant subtest as an early indicator of cognitive decline related to DAD in people with DS.

Although the SIB was not specifically designed for people with ID, preliminary studies in this population appear to show that it is a potentially useful instrument to assess cognitive decline in conditions, such as DS. Like many other neuropsychometric assessments; however, it is necessary that the participant retains some SIB in Witts and Elders study[65] was probable due to the relatively high functioning sample. The test is unlikely to be useful for people with profound ID or severe dementia.

Cambridge Cognitive Examination

The CAMCOG is part of the Cambridge Examination for Mental Disorders of the Elderly-Revised (CAMDEX-R).[14,66] The CAMDEX is a diagnostic assessment that provides a means to identify dementia and to differentiate it from other common disorders and the normal processes of aging developed for the general population.[14] The CAMDEX-R is the revised and updated version of the CAMDEX[66] enabling a clinical diagnosis of dementia to be made on the basis of internationally agreed criteria (e.g., DSM-IV, ICD-10). The CAMCOG is a concise group of neuropsychological tests covering all areas of cognitive function that characteristically decline with the onset of dementia. The MMSE[56] is also contained in the CAMCOG and can be used to obtain a global estimate of ability.

Data are collected within the CAMDEX-R through structured clinical interview of an informant supplying systematic information about the presenting disorder, past and family history, present state and history. The CAMCOG is administered by a qualified clinician such as a psychiatrist, psychologist, geriatrician, epidemiologist, or other mental health professional working within psychiatry for the elderly. The evaluator works directly with the person being assessed using verbal and visual stimulus items. These items relate to subscales for orientation, language, memory, praxis, attention/calculation, abstract thinking and perception, thus giving subscales scores and a total score.

The CAMDEX-R and CAMCOG have been used with some modifications in adults with DS.[28,29,67,68] These authors concluded that the modified CAMCOG was useful to assess areas of cognitive function known to decline with dementia in persons with DS. However, person with preexisting severe ID, severe sensory impairments, and/or already advanced dementia may not be able to score above the "floor level" of the test.[28]

Although the modified CAMCOG has shown to promising results in high functioning people with DS, giving its length and level of complexity, it is unlikely to be able to be used successfully in the majority of people with DS. The CAMDEX and CAMCOG have not yet been validated to permit a clinical differentiation of the various types of dementia.[67] Additionally, studies examining the early detection of dementia in persons in the general population have suggested that CAMCOG scores are affected by age, hearing and visual defects (e.g., decreased visual acuity and contrast sensitivity due to cataracts).[69,70]

The Dyspraxia Scale

The Dyspraxia scale (Chapter 5) was developed by Dalton and Fedor in 1998.[71] Dyspraxia is a partial loss of ability to perform purposeful or skilled motor actions in the absence of paralysis, sensory loss, abnormal posture or tone, abnormal involuntary movements, lack of coordination, poor comprehension or inattention.[72] The Dyspraxia scale is an instrument that provides a tool for the evaluation of simple sequences of movements without requiring a normal level of verbal comprehension or communication skills that are found in persons with learning disability.[41,73] It is not a test of cognitive abilities per se, in fact it does not attempt to assess language or comprehension skills. Its use is based on the premise that praxis is expected to deteriorate with the onset and progress of dementia in people with mild to profound ID. The test has 62 items and directly assesses the ability of a person to perform short sequences of voluntary movements such as walking, clapping, etc. The authors reported good test–retest reliability ($r = .96$) item by item reliability ($\alpha = .97$) predictive and face validity but noticed that the validity has not been established against neuropathological diagnoses.[71] It has been used in research with community-based populations of people with ID.[74]

The Adaptive Behavior Dementia Questionnaire

The Adaptive Behavior Dementia Questionnaire (ABDQ; Chapter 10) was developed by Prasher and colleagues in 2004[75] as a screening questionnaire for DAD in adults with DS. It was based on the analysis of 5-year consecutive data changes on part I of the Adaptive Behavior Scale[36] as part of an ongoing annual thorough assessment of adults with DS. For the development of the ABDQ, 150 adults with DS (mean age 44.0 ± 1.46, range 16–76) were assessed on baseline by review of previously reported intelligence tests, previous level of functioning as determined by review of medical notes, from carer interview and from the mental state examination; severity of the ID was classified using ICD-10 criteria.[1] All persons were followed up on an annual basis as part of ongoing clinical care with detailed reassessments of their physical and mental health, adaptive behavior, and social needs. Findings for the absence or presence of DAD were compared to changes in the ABS measurements over the 5 years follow up to determine which items of the ABS best correlated with deterioration in intellectual functioning and could be subsequently used to develop a screening questionnaire.

The ABDQ is a brief questionnaire with good validity and interrater reliability that screens for DAD specifically and not just dementia per se. The ABDQ has been developed from over 10 years of research investigating changes in adaptive behavior in adults with DS. It can be used for all adults with ID irrespective of ID and severity of DAD. Once the baseline level of independent functioning of a particular person has been established with the full ABS, the ABDQ appears to be a useful instrument for the ongoing assessment of people with DS. The instrument may prove to be of value as a tool to assess treatment response in drug trials and to monitor changes over time without having to repeat the full lengthy and time-consuming ABS itself.

However, given the heterogeneity on presentation on the early stages of dementia and the relative sparse information about behavioral changes associated with the early stages of DAD in this population it is difficult to assume that a individual patient will fit on any of the behavioral categories included in the ABDQ. Individual clinicians may need to rely on changes identified in the full ABS questionnaire to identify decline and monitor illness progression rather than the ABDQ. In any case, although behavioral changes are part of the presentation of dementia, such changes of behavior on their own cannot be used to screen for dementia (whether in people with ID on in the general population). Diagnosis of dementia requires a fuller clinical assessment together with a mixture of direct assessments of cognitive abilities, informant-based history, and exclusion of other causes of behavioral changes.

The Prudhoe Cognitive Function Test

The Prudhoe Cognitive Function Test (PCFT) was designed by Kay and colleagues in 1985,[76] but not published until 2003,[77] for the direct assessment of cognitive abilities in people with DS. This test can be used by clinicians and other health professionals, not only by psychologists. It was intended to detect cognitive decline over time, to be used serially and therefore not as a single use diagnostic tool. The PCFT is based on subjects' direct responses, and avoids relying on carers' memories and perceptions of the subject's ability. Administration of the PCFT takes no more than 35 min. It covers the major domains of cognitive functioning which are usually examined when testing or screening normal adults for dementia, i.e., orientation, recall, language, praxis, and calculation, some of which are divided into further subdomains. At the end of the PCFT, the interviewer rates speech, hearing, and vision on ad hoc four-point scales, from normal, through mild and severe, to profound impairment. Two shorter versions of the PCFT, Form A and Form B, that only take less than 15 min to administer, have now been developed. The correlations between these short versions of the PCFT and the long version was found to be extremely high at 0.97 for Form A and 0.98 for Form B, illustrating that both short forms and the long form are essentially interchangeable.[78]

Reliability

To assess the interrater and test–retest reliability of the PCFT, three raters (the researcher and two fourth-year medical students), administered the tests to 14 adults with DS without dementia on two occasions, 4 weeks apart. The intraclass correlation coefficient (ICC) in both the interrater (ICC = 0.99, $p = 0.01$) and test–retest reliability (ICC = 0.99, $p = 0.01$) measures were very high, showing that the PCFT is a highly reliable instrument with excellent temporal stability.

Validity

The PCFT has been validated against the Kaufman Brief Intelligence Test (K-BIT),[79] a standardized instrument that has been utilized widely to assess cognitive abilities in people with ID. Comparison of performance on the long PCFT in 167 subjects with equal representation of mild, moderate, and severe ID showed high correlations between the verbal and performance sections of the K-BIT with correlation coefficients of 0.85 and 0.78, respectively.[78] The results of the different domains of the

PCFT parallel these correlations with K-BIT vocabulary, which, with the exception of recall, ranged between .77 (language) and .85 (both praxis and calculation). These same PCFT domains correlate similarly with the nonverbal component of the K-BIT. The correlations range between .71 (orientation and language) and .80 (praxis). As with the correlations between each short form and the long form, the correlations for the recall domain were the lowest. This suggests that the items comprising this domain are more difficult to score reliably than is true of the remaining four PCFT domains. This receives support from the results of the Margallo-Lana and colleagues[77] investigation in which the overall reliability was excellent (.99). However, the only domains not to be scored in the good (.60–.74) to excellent range (.75–1.00) were immediate and delayed recall (<.40). Examination of the items in this domain showed that there was ambiguity in the order of asking the questions concerned and problems arose in subjects who were temporally orientated and so further questions regarding time concepts were not able to test verbal recall in these individuals. These issues are addressed below.

The PCFT has face validity in terms of the acceptability of test items to both user and subjects. It also has content validity as the test questions are representative of the skills in the specified domains of the test. Most of the items were chosen on the basis of knowledge of dementia in people without ID. For example, the items concerning naming objects and obeying simple requests are similar to questions used in standard neuropsychiatry examination of dementia such as the MMSE.[56]

Other forms of validity such as predictive validity (whether it adequately predicts performance), construct validity (whether it measures the right psychological constructs), or criterion validity (whether it correlates with existing tests which purport to measure the same construct) still need to be assessed. Its validity as an aid to diagnosing dementia in mental retardation is being evaluated in the Prudhoe longitudinal study by correlating its longitudinal performance with the clinical and pathological data. In the latest results of this investigation a dementia diagnosis in all patients was accompanied by a global decline in all the five domains of the PCFT.[80]

Specificity and Sensitivity

The sensitivity and specificity of the PCFT as an instrument to assess cognitive decline associated with dementia needs to be established. Information gained during the ongoing follow-up of the original cohort for whom it was initially developed will help to assess these psychometric properties.

Down Syndrome Attention, Memory, and Executive Function Scales (DAMES)

The DAMES is a battery developed for the assessment of attention, memory, and executive function in people with DS.(80) The tests included in the DAMES were drawn from a large battery of neuropsychological tests used on a cross-sectional controlled study about age-related neuropsychological changes in 122 adults with DS.[80] The rationale for developing the original battery of tests was based on recent literature pertaining to early symptoms of DAD in the general population. The literature in this subject suggests that apart from the episodic memory deficits that are crucial feature in DAD, attentional and executive function dysfunction are present in the disease at an early stage.[73,81] There are very few tests to specifically assess attention, executive function, and memory in adults with learning disabilities (particularly the first two areas). Thus, the development of a battery "de novo" for this population that borrowed tests specifically designed to assess adults and children in the general population was thought to provide a comprehensive tool. The advantages of using these as part of the DAME scales are that these are well-established tests with known profiles of performance and that they are likely to show little floor effect in the people with ID.

The tests included in the DAMES were selected from those tests on the larger battery that were sensitive to change on the test performance over a year and able to differentiate between participants with DS above and below 40 years of age. The tests included in the DAMES involve tests of attention, memory, and executive function. Attention tests include tests of (1) focused attention or concentration,[82] which refers to the ability to highlight one or two important stimuli while suppressing awareness of competing distractions and (2) selective attention, the ability to respond to specific stimuli and screen out irrelevant stimuli.[83] Both forms of attention have been shown to be defective in the early stages of DAD in the general population.[73] Tests of executive function are also included. Executive function (problem solving, adapting strategies, and judgment) is also disrupted in the early stages of DAD,[84] so tests to assess this function were also included as well as test of memory, both visual and auditory.

The performance on 11 tests from the original battery was sensitive to change over a year and differentiated persons with DS below and above the age of 40 years.[80] People with DS aged 40 years and over without dementia experienced a decline of 11% over 1 year, indicating that progressive cognitive decline precedes dementia (and hence offers an important opportunity for prevention) and that these measurements are sensitive to cognitive change over time in this group of older people with DS. This degree of progression of cognitive impairment is comparable to the annual rate of decline in people with DAD in the general population. As virtually all people with DS aged 40 years and over have evidence of AD in the brain, it would be expected that they should experience progressive cognitive decline, even if a formal arbitrary diagnosis of clinical dementia has not been made. The range of scores is 0–222.

Reliability

The interrater and test–retest reliability of the DAMES has been assessed by two psychologist on a group of adults with DS with and without dementia and it has been shown to be very good (intraclass correlation coefficient above .90 in both instance, Margallo-Lana et al., unpublished study).

Validity

The validity of the DAMES is being assessed as part of an international drug trial study in people with DS and without dementia. The DAMES scores will be correlated with the K-BIT[79]: a brief, reliable, and validated individually administered test of verbal and nonverbal intelligence.

Summary

When diagnosing dementia in adults with ID, the most important consideration is that the diagnosis requires a change in status. Longitudinal assessments that document baseline cognitive functioning, in addition to a change in independent functioning, are necessary before sufficient information can be obtained to make a diagnosis of dementia.[5] However, as in the general population, it is not sufficient to identify decline in cognitive and functional skills to conclude that a person suffers from dementia as other causes of apparent decline must be excluded before a confident diagnosis can be made. The perception of decline will also depend on the environmental demands on the individual.[3]

As in the general population, the results of any test are meaningless if considered in isolation without its clinical context. In people with severe and profound ID, who usually fall outside the lower range of scores of most available instruments, assessment of cognitive and behavioral skills may not be possible and one may have to rely on other aspects of the history and presentation, such as development of neurological symptoms (epilepsy or dysphagia). Equally, in the general population, people with very high intellectual skills may not be correctly identified as decline in performance in common tests used for screening of dementia in the general population such as the MMSE[56] rely on subtle changes in behavior identified on clinical assessment, rather than on psychometric test scores.

It may be advisable in the future to abandon the use of a single instrument that attempts to diagnose dementia in this population and accept that we need to use an array of assessments to fully understand the nature of the process that is affecting that individual. An early diagnosis of whether a person is suffering from dementia will aid not only the individual but also the carers and people in contact with the individual to understand and adapt to the changes that will inevitably accompanied the illness.

References

1. World Health Organisation (1992). The ICD-10 Classification of Mental and Behavioural Disorders. Geneva: World Health Organisation.
2. American Psychiatric Association (1994). Diagnostic and Statistical Manual of Mental Disorders, 4th edn. Washington, DC: APA.

3. Aylward E, Burt D, and Thorpe L et al. (1997). Diagnosis of dementia in individuals with intellectual disability. J Intellect Disabil Res 36: 337–347.
4. Thompson S (1999). Examining dementia in Down syndrome (DS): Decline in social abilities in DS compared with other learning disabilities. Clin Geronto 20: 23–44.
5. Burt DB and Aylward EH (1998). Test battery for the Diagnosis of Dementia in Individuals with Intellectual Disability. Washington, DC: American Association of Mental Retardation.
6. Harper D and Wadsworth J (1993). A primer on dementia in persons with mental retardation: Conclusions and current findings. In: Dosen RFA, editor. Mental Health Aspects of Mental Retardation. New York: Lexington Books.
7. Geyde A (1995). Manual for the Dementia Scale for Down Syndrome. Vancouver, Canada: Geyde Research and Consulting.
8. Burt D and Aylward E (1999). Assessment methods for diagnosis of dementia. In: Dalton MJA, editor. Dementia, Aging and Intellectual Disabilities. New York: Brunner/Mazel.
9. Thompson S (2001). Assessing dementia in Down's syndrome: A comparison of five tests. Clin Geronto 23: 3-19.
10. Evenhuis HM, Kengen MMF, and Eurlings HAL (1990). Dementia Questionnaire for Mentally Retarded Persons. Zwammerdam, the Netherlands: Hooge Burch.
11. Albert M and Cohen C (1992). The test for severe impairment: An instrument for the assessment of patients with severe cognitive dysfunction. J Am Geriatr Soc 40: 449-453.
12. Saxton J, McGonigle-Gibson K, and Swihart A et al. (1990). Assessment of the severely impaired patient: Description and validation of a new neuropsychological test battery psychological assessment. J Consult Clin Psychol 2: 298-303.
13. Strydom A and Hassiotis A (2003). Diagnostic instruments for dementia in older people with intellectual disability in clinical practice. Aging Ment Health 6: 431-437.
14. Roth M, Tym E, and Mountjoy CQ (1986). CAMDEX–A standardised instrument for the diagnosis of mental disorder in the elderly with special reference to the early detection of dementia. Br J Psychiatry 149: 698-709.
15. Wilson B, Cockburn J, and Baddeley A (1985). The Rivermead Behavioural Memory Test. Flempton: Thames Valley Test Company.
16. Wilson B, Ivani Chalian R, and Aldrich F (1991). The Rivermead Behavioural Memory Test for Children Aged 5-10. Suffolk: Thames Valley.
17. Wechsler D (1997). Wechsler Adult Intelligence Scales, 3rd edn. San Antonio, TX: The Psychological Corporation.
18. Raven J, Court J, and Raven J (1995). Raven Manual: Section 2. Coloured Progressive Matrices 1995 Edition. Oxford: Oxford Psychologists Press.
19. Golding E (1989). The Middlesex Elderly Assessment of Mental State. Bury St. Edmunds: Thames Valley Test Company.
20. HSS-Hampshire Social Services. (1989). Hampshire Social Services Assessment. Southampton: Hampshire Social Services.
21. Cosgrave MP, McCarron M, Anderson M et al. (1998). Cognitive decline in Down syndrome: a validity/reliability study of the test for severe impairment. Am J Ment Retard 103: 193-197.
22. Nelson L, Lott I, Touchette P, et al. (1995). Detection of Alzheimer's disease in individuals with Down syndrome. Am J Ment Retard 99: 616-622.
23. Prasher V, Krishnan V, Clarke D et al. (1994). The assessment of dementia in people with Down syndrome: Changes in adaptive behaviour. Br J Develop Disabil 90: 120-130.
24. Visser F and Kuilman M (1990). A study of dementia in Down's syndrome of an institutionalised population. Nederlands Tijdschrift voor Geneeskunde 134: 1141-1145.
25. Evenhuis H (1992). Evaluation of a screening instrument for dementia in ageing mentally retarded persons. J Intellect Disabil Res 36: 337-347.
26. Zelinski E and Gilewski M (1998). Assessment of memory complaints by rating scales and questionnaires. Psychopharma Bull 24: 523-529.
27. Shultz J, Aman M, Kelbley T et al. (2004). Evaluation of screening tools for dementia in older adults with mental retardation. Am J Ment Retard 2: 98-110.

28. Hon J, Huppert FA, Holland AJ et al. (1999). Neuropsychological assessment of older adults with Down syndrome: An epidemiological study using the Cambridge Cognitive Examination (CAMCOG). Br J Clin Psychol 38: 155-165.
29. Holland AJ, Hon J, Huppert FA et al. (2000). Incidence and course of dementia in people with Down's syndrome: Findings from a population-based study. J Intellect Disabil Res 44: 138-146.
30. National Institute for Health and Clinical Excellence-Social Care Institute for Excellence NICE-SCIE, Guideline to improve care of people with dementia, November 2006.
31. Seltzer G (1997). Modified Fuld Object Memory Evaluation. , Madison, WI: Waisman Centre, University of Wisconsin Madison.
32. Kaplan E, Goodglass H, and Weubtraub S (1983). The Boston Naming Test. Philadelphia, PA: Lea & Febiger.
33. McCarthy D (1972). Manual for the McCarthy Scales of Children's Ability. San Antonio, TX: The Psychological Corporation.
34. Haxby JV (1989). Neuropsychological evaluation of adults with Down syndrome: Patterns of selective impairment in adults non-demented old adults. J Ment Defic Res 33: 193-210.
35. Tiffin J and Asher E (1984). The Purdue Pegboard: Norms and studies and validity. J Appl Psychol 32: 234-247.
36. Nihira K, Foster R, Shellhaas M et al. (1974). Adaptive Behavior Scale. Washington, DC: American Association on Mental Retardation.
37. Prasher V (1998). Adaptive behavior. In: Janicki MP and Dalton AJ, editors. Dementia, Aging, and Intellectual Disabilities. Philadelphia, PA: Taylor & Francis, pp. 157-178.
38. Zigman W, Schupf N, Lubin R et al. (1987). Premature regression of adults with Down syndrome. Am J Ment Defic 92: 161-168.
39. Devenny D, Silverman W, Hill A, et al. (1996). Normal ageing in adults with Down syndrome: A longitudinal study. J Intellect Disabil Res 40: 208-221.
40. Visser FE, Aldenkamp AP, HuffelenAC, et al. (1997). Prospective study of the prevalence of Alzheimer type dementia in institutionalised individuals with Down syndrome. Am J Ment Retard 101: 400-412.
41. Dalton A and Fedor B (1997). The multi-dimensional observation scale for elderly subjects applied for persons with Down syndrome. In: Proceedings of the International Congress III on the Dually Diagnosed, National Association for the Dually Diagnosed, Washington, DC, pp. 173-178.
42. Evenhuis HM (1992). Provisional Manual of the Dementia Questionnaire for Mentally Retarded Persons (DMR). Zwammerdam, the Netherlands: Hooge Burch.
43. Evenhuis HM, Eurlings HAL, and Kengen MMF (1984). Diagnostiek van dementia bijbejaarde zwakzinnigen (diagnosis of dementia in mentally retarded persons). Ruit 40: 14-24.
44. Evenhuis H (1996). Further evaluation of the Dementia Questionnaire for Persons with Mental Retardation (DMR). J Intellect Disabil Res 40: 369-373.
45. Evenhuis HM (1990). The natural history of dementia in Down's syndrome. Arch Neurol 47: 263-267.
46. Thompson SBN (1994). A neuropsychological test battery for identifying dementia in people with Down syndrome. Br J Devel Disabil XL; 2: 135-142.
47. Prasher V (1997). Dementia questionnaire for persons with mental retardation (DMR): Modified criteria for adults with Down syndrome. J Appl Res Intellect Disabil 10: 54-60.
48. Deb S and Braganza J (1999). Comparison of rating scales for the diagnosis of dementia in adults with Down syndrome. J Intellect Disabil Res 43: 400-407.
49. Aylward E and Burt D (1998). Test battery for the diagnosis of dementia in individuals with intellectual disability. Report of the Working Group for the Establishment of Criteria for the Diagnosis of Dementia in Individuals with Intellectual Disability. Washington, DC: American Association on Mental Retardation.
50. Deb S, Braganza J, Norton N et al. (1998). No significant association between a PS-1 intronic polymorphism and dementia in Down syndrome. Alzheimer's Report 1: 365-368.
51. Hoekman J and Maaskant MA (2002). Comparison of instruments for the diagnosis of dementia in individuals with intellectual disability. J Intellect Dev Disabil 27: 296-309.

52. Jorm AF (1994). A short form of the Informant Questionnaire on Cognitive Decline in the Elderly (IQCODE): Development and cross-validation. Psychol Med 24: 145-145.
53. Schultz JM, Aman MG, and Rojahn J (1998). Psychometric evaluation of a measure of cognitive decline in elderly people with mental retardation. Res Develop Disabil 19: 63-71.
54. Cosgrave MP, Tyrell J, McCarron M et al. (2000). A five year follow-up study of dementia in persons with Down syndrome: Early symptoms and pattern of deterioration. Ir J Psychol Med 17: 5-11.
55. Oliver C (1999). Perspectives on assessment and evaluation. In: Dalton MJA, editor. Dementia, Ageing and Intellectual Disabilities. New York: Brunner/Maze.
56. Folstein M, Folstein S, and McHugh P (1975). Mini-mental state: A practical method of grading the cognitive state of patients for the clinician. J Psychiatr Res 12: 189-198.
57. Sturmey P, Reed J, and Corbett J (1991). Psychometric assessment of psychiatric disorders in people with learning difficulties (mental handicap): A review of measures. Psychol Med 21: 143-155.
58. Aylward E, Burt D, Thorpe L et al. (1995). Diagnosis of Dementia in Individuals with Intellectual Disability. Washington, DC: American Association of Mental Retardation.
59. Tyrell J, Cosgrave M, McLaughlin M et al. (1996). Dementia in an Irish population of Down syndrome people. Ir J Psychol Med 13: 51-54.
60. Pippi M, Mecocci P, Saxton J et al. (1999). Neuropsychological assessment of the severely impaired elderly patient: Validation of the Italian short version of the Severe Impairment Battery (SIB). Gruppo di Studio sull'Invecchiamento Cerebrale della Societa Italiana di Gerontologia e Geriatria. Aging (Milano) 11: 221-226.
61. Llinas RJ, Lozano GM, Lopez OL et al. (1995). Validation of the Spanish version of the Severe Impairment Battery. Neurologia 10: 14-18 (in Spanish).
62. Panisset M, Roudier M, Saxton J et al. (1992) A battery of neuropsychological tests for severe dementia. An evaluation study. Presse Med 21: 1271-1274 (in French).
63. McKenzie K, Harte C, Sinclair E et al.(2002). An examination of the Severe Impairment Battery as a measure of cognitive decline in clients with Down's syndrome. J Learn Disabil 6: 89-96.
64. Prasher VP, Huxley A, and Haque MS (2002). Down syndrome ageing study group A 24-week, double-blind, placebo-controlled trial of donepezil in patients with Down syndrome and Alzheimer's disease-Pilot study. Int J Geriatr Psychiatry 17: 270-278.
65. Witts P and Elders S (1998). The Severe Impairment Battery: Assessing cognitive ability in adults with Down syndrome. Br J Clin Psychol 37: 13-16.
66. Roth M, Huppert FA, Mountjoy CQ et al. (1998). CAMDEX-R The Cambridge Examination. Cambridge: Cambridge University Press.
67. Holland AJ, Hon J, Huppert FA et al. (1998). Population-based study of the prevalence and presentation of dementia in adults with Down's syndrome. Br J Psychiatry 172: 493-498.
68. Ball SL, Holland AJ, Huppert FA et al. (2004). The modified CAMDEX informant interview is a valid and reliable tool for use in the diagnosis of dementia in adults with Down's syndrome. J Intellect Disabil Res 48: 611-620.
69. Blessed G, Black SE, Butler T et al. (1991). The diagnosis of dementia in the elderly: A comparison of CAMCOG (the cognitive section of CAMDEX), the AGECAT Program, DSM-III, the Mini-Mental State Examination and some short rating scales. Br J Psychiatry 159: 193–198.
70. Hartman JA (2000). Investigation of the use of the CAMCOG in the visually impaired. Int J Geriatr Psychiatry 15: 863-869.
71. Dalton A and Fedor B (1998). Onset of dyspraxia in aging persons with Down syndrome: Longitudinal studies. J Intellect Dev Disabil Res 23: 13–24.
72. Lohr J and Wisniewski A (1987). Movement Disorders: A Neuropsychiatric Approach. New York: Guilford Press.
73. Perry R and Hodges R (1999). Attention and executive deficits in Alzheimer's disease: A critical review. Brain 122: 383-404.
74. Dalton AJ, Sano MC, and Aisen PS (2001). Brief Praxis test: A primary outcome measure for treatment trial of Alzheimer disease in persons with Down syndrome. Multi-centre Vitamin E

trial: Project proposal. New York: New York State Institute for Basic Research in Developmental Disabilities.

75. Prasher VP, Farooq A, and Holder R (2004). The Adaptive Behaviour Dementia Questionnaire (ABDQ): Screening Questionnaire for dementia of Alzheimer's disease in adults with Down syndrome. Res Develop Disabil 25: 385-397.

76. Kay DW, Tyrer SP, Margallo-Lana et al. (2003). The Prudhoe Cognitive Function scale to assess cognitive function in adults with Down's syndrome: Inter-rater and test-retest reliability. J Intellect Disabil Res 47:488-492.

77. Margallo-Lana ML, Moore P, Tyrer S et al. (2003). The Prudhoe Cognitive Function Test: A scale to assess function in adults with Down's syndrome. Inter-rater and test-retest reappraisal. J Intellect Dev Disabil Res 47: 488-492.

78. Reid BE, Wigham A, Cicchetti DV et al. (2005). A comparison of two forms of the Prudhoe Cognitive Function Test with the Kaufman Brief Intelligence Test (K-BIT) In: Corretger JM, Sers A, Casaldliga J, and Trias K, editors. Sndrome de Down. Aspectos mdicos actuales. Barcelona: Masson, pp. 384-385.

79. Kaufman AS and Kaufman NL (1990). Kaufman Brief Intelligence Test Manual (K-BIT). Circle Pines, MN: American Guidance Service.

80. Margallo-Lana, M, Moore PB, Kay DWK et al. (2007). 15-year follow up of 92 hospitalised adults with Down's Syndrome: Relationship of cognitive decline to neurofibrillary tangle count. J Intellect Disabil Res 51: 463-477.

81. Baddeley A, Baddeley H, Buchks R et al. (2001). Attentional control in Alzheimer's disease. Brain 124: 1479-1481.

82. Nebes R and Brady C (1989). Focused and divided attention in Alzheimer's disease. Cortex 25: 305-315.

83. Sohlberg M and Mateer C (1989). Introduction to Cognitive Rehabilitation. New York: Guilford Press.

84. Grady CL, Haxby JV, Horwitz B et al. (1988). Longitudinal study of the early neuropsychological and cerebral metabolic changes in dementia of the Alzheimer type. J Clin Exp Neuropsychol 10: 576-596.

Chapter 2
Issues in Dementia Assessment Methods

D.B. Burt

Introduction

Dementia assessment in adults with intellectual disabilities (ID) is a challenging task, but recent work by clinicians and researchers has improved diagnostic accuracy. Diagnostic criteria were outlined[1] and found to be feasible and useful.[2–4] A battery of tests was proposed to identify declines needed to meet diagnostic criteria.[5,6] Ongoing investigations examined the sensitivity and specificity of tests from the proposed battery and additional alternative batteries.[2,3,7–20] The purpose of this chapter is to outline and discuss general issues and factors that can affect dementia assessment either directly or indirectly.[3,8] Such issues are important to consider when evaluating tests for clinical and research purposes. As indicated in Table 2.1, a discussion of general theoretical issues will be followed by a more specific discussion of methodological issues.

Worldview Implications: Adults with Down Syndrome

Historically, clinicians and researchers approached the assessment of dementia in adults with Down syndrome (DS) from two worldviews.[21] The first assumes that all adults with DS get dementia in Alzheimer's disease (DAD). Changes in functioning starting around age 30 years are assumed to be early dementia.[22,23] The second world view, in contrast, assumes that only some adults with DS get dementia. Declines in functioning are not always indicative of dementia, particularly dementia of DAD.[21,24] As in the general population, it is assumed that declines could be due to multiple infarcts,[25–27] conditions like Parkinson's disease,[28] adverse drug effects,[29] or other psychiatric disorders (e.g., depression).[30–32]

Although clinicians and researchers do not always explicitly state their adopted worldview, it has an effect on the evaluation and use of assessment scales. According to the first worldview, the purpose of dementia assessment is to detect declines related to dementia and to illustrate the natural history of dementia. If declines are not eventually detected on a given scale, the scale is assumed not to be sensitive

V.P. Prasher (ed.), *Neuropsychological Assessments of Dementia in Down Syndrome and Intellectual Disabilities*,
DOI: 10.1007/978-1-84800-249-4_2, © Springer Science+Business Media, LLC 2009

Table 2.1 Issues in Dementia Assessment

Worldview implications	Adults with Down syndrome and Alzheimer's disease
Schedule of assessment	Single versus repeated evaluations
Purpose of assessment	Diagnosis, declines identified, screening, differential diagnosis
Characteristics of individuals being assessed	Intellectual level, age, etiology of ID, gender
Methods to address individual differences	Homogeneous versus stratified samples
Source of information	Informant report versus direct assessment of performance
Evaluation of assessment scales and techniques	Independent/external criterion, measures (sensitivity, specificity, predictive value), reliability, group comparisons, stages of dementia, strength/weakness profiles, clinical usefulness

enough. Advocates of the second worldview use assessment scales to differentiate clinically significant declines from those associated with typical aging. They also attempt to differentiate declines associated with irreversible dementia from those associated with other treatable conditions (e.g., depression). The recent focus on standardized diagnostic criteria is designed to maximize diagnostic accuracy and to minimize the number of adults erroneously diagnosed with DAD.[1,22]

Other theoretical assumptions related to one's adopted worldview also influence assessment. If, for example, one assumes that all adults with DS get DAD and show the same sequence of decline (e.g., memory decline followed by motor decline,[9] dyspraxia followed by other cognitive decline[33]), then tests for memory decline or dyspraxia could be adopted to screen for early signs of dementia. Any adult who showed early signs of dementia in another area (e.g., changes in emotional functioning[2,7,8]) would not be identified by a narrow screening battery assessing only memory or dyspraxia. Similarly, if one assumes that all adults with DS or with other forms of ID get only a progressive dementia like that caused by DAD,[1] then an adult who shows signs of a static dementia (e.g., related to adverse effects of medication) may not be identified. Whether or not all adults with DS or with other forms of ID get DAD, and when they do whether they show the same invariant sequence of declines are issues currently being investigated. In the meantime, effects of worldview on assessment in individual cases and in general must be considered in order to minimize diagnostic error (e.g., in research).

Schedule for Assessment

When considering dementia assessment scales, it is necessary to examine the intended schedule and purpose of the scale. Regarding scheduling, a scale or test battery can be developed for a single administration, with performance at that one assessment presumed to be indicative of dementia status. An example of such a scale used in the general population is the Mini-Mental State Examination.[34] If an adult performs below a certain cutoff point on this scale at one assessment, they are assumed to be demented. The use of single-administration scales with adults with ID is complicated by the fact that low performance is likely to be related to level of ID and not to dementia.[3,8,16]

Other single-administration scales rely on retrospective reporting, like the Dementia Scale for Down Syndrome (DSDS; Chapter 4).[35] On this scale, informants are asked to compare current behavior to remembered behavior. Although the scale is also used at repeated assessments, dementia status is based on absolute scores not on change scores, which indicate differences between current and previous performance. The advantage of such single-administration scales is the practicality of determining dementia status at one assessment. The disadvantage is that performance can be confounded by level of ID and by inaccuracies in retrospective reporting.

Scales can also be developed to allow direct comparisons of performance across repeated assessments. Declines in performance over time are then examined to see if they correspond to clinically significant changes indicative of dementia. Scales and tests in the battery recommended by the dementia work group,[5,6] for example, were intended for repeated assessment, with baseline performance compared to later performance. Scales have also been developed for use both at one assessment and across repeated assessments. The Dementia Questionnaire for People with Intellectual Disabilities (DMR; Chapter 3), for example, had both a scoring system for a single administration and a system for examining change scores that reflected differences in scores over repeated assessments.[36] The advantage of such a dual scoring system is that dementia status can be determined at one assessment, thus alerting the evaluator to the need for a further dementia workup.[37] The scale can also be administered repeatedly to gather further evidence about dementia status and progression. Interestingly, the two scoring systems yielded differences in sensitivity and specificity to dementia.[3,16,38] Most recently, Evenhuis and colleagues recommended use of repeated assessments only. They no longer recommend single administration of the scale.[39,40]

Purpose of Assessment

The advantage of single versus repeated assessments is related to the purpose of a scale or test battery. Clinicians and investigators have developed scales for different purposes. A broad battery of tests may be used repeatedly, for example, to determine whether diagnostic criteria for dementia are met (i.e., memory decline, other cognitive decline, changes in emotional functioning, declines in everyday functioning). In such a battery, multiple scales are included on the basis of each scale's ability to detect declines related to a given diagnostic criterion.[3,8] A sentence recall task, for example, is administered to assess declines in memory, whereas a vocabulary test is included to assess declines in cognition, specifically language. An advantage of a broad battery, in addition to allowing assessment of all areas needed for dementia diagnosis, is that the clinician or researcher can examine combinations of tests and scales to see which subsets of tests lead to the greatest levels of sensitivity and specificity.[3,8,16] In addition, when tests are administered repeatedly, performance can be examined to see if some tests detect earlier signs of dementia and thus would serve as useful screens for dementia at one assessment.[3,8,41–46] Performance can also be examined to see if other tests detect later signs of dementia and thus would serve best as repeated measures over time for confirmation of the presence of dementia.[3,8]

In contrast, researchers and clinicians have designed broad scales, assessing several areas of functioning, to repeatedly assess all areas needed for dementia diagnosis.[2,36,39,40] Performance on the scale is compared to other tests designed to independently determine dementia status. If one scale can diagnose dementia as accurately as a more extensive battery, then the single scale could be more efficient and cost-effective. The sensitivity and specificity of such a broad scale would need to be determined.

Test batteries have also been used with a narrower focus, for example, to detect declines on tests of memory and other cognitive functioning.[41–46] In such cases, an external criterion for dementia is needed to relate performance on the scale to dementia status to determine the test's usefulness in dementia assessment. Others have examined performance on one scale assessing a single skill (e.g., dyspraxia) to examine declines in functioning related to an intervention (e.g., with vitamin E) without necessarily relating the declines to actual dementia status.[14,33] Such scales would also require an external criterion for dementia to determine relationships between performance and dementia status.

In examining the purpose of scales and instruments, it is necessary to examine any rationale given for the schedule of assessment (one administration, repeated administrations, both types of administration). It is advantageous to know whether a scale is useful in early detection of dementia, in the confirmation of dementia status, or perhaps both. A screening instrument for early detection would ideally be less time-consuming and less expensive, so that it could be administered repeatedly without using vast amounts of scarce recourses. Screening scales also need to provide information in a format easily integrated into an adult's permanent record, because screening or baseline data are only useful if they can be located easily and compared to later performance. Such screening instruments could be administered when the adult is known to be functioning optimally (e.g., young adulthood), with repeated administrations designed to determine a pattern of functioning for the individual.[3,8] The screening instrument would then be readministered periodically or sooner if dementia is suspected.

A test or battery of tests designed to allow a confirmation that dementia diagnostic criteria are met will by definition need to be more comprehensive. To be useful, such a battery would also need to be administered at least once when an adult is known to be healthy to allow for later comparisons to baseline functioning.[1] Such a battery or broad test will also need to contain aspects that allow for differential diagnosis of dementia from other psychiatric disorders such as depression, medical conditions such as thyroid disease, or adverse drug effects.[7,10,31,32,47–56] It may not be feasible to administer such a broad battery or test on a regular schedule, because of scarce resources.

Characteristics of Individuals Being Assessed

Characteristics of individuals such as level of functioning (usually intellectual level given as intelligence quotient (IQ) or mild, moderate, severe), age, cause of ID, and gender have all been shown to influence test performance.[3,8,16,58] For healthy adults, such individual differences influence performance at one assessment and also affect the amount of change over time that is typical. When examining assessment instruments, therefore, one should determine what considerations were made for individual characteristics (e.g., cutoff scores for dementia calculated by level of functioning, change scores indicative of significant decline adjusted for age[27]). It is also necessary to determine the characteristics of the standardization sample to see for whom a test or scale is designed.

Intellectual Level

General reasoning as indicated by IQ was related to performance on almost all tests such that higher IQ is related to higher performance.[3,8,16,58] Level of functioning was also related to change in performance over time. Adults at lower levels of functioning showed improvements in performance with repeated practice, whereas higher functioning adults started at a higher level and remained at the same level.[21] Thus, amount and type of change in performance over time can be related to initial level of functioning, which would need to be considered in differentiating typical performance from that associated with dementia. Dementia cutoff scores based on informant reports, such as those on the original single administration of the DMR,[36] also require adjustment for premorbid level of functioning (i.e., when healthy). The challenges in making such adjustments are that methods for assessing level of functioning change over an adult's life span (e.g., as intelligence tests are revised), different tests are used for a given adult across time often yielding vastly different results (e.g., Weschler versus Stanford–Binet tests), and methods are not standard across countries.[16]

Age

If a skill is influenced by aging, then one would expect the amount of decline over time that is typical for healthy, older adults to be different from that of healthy, younger adults. Different criteria could be needed for adults of different ages, therefore, to indicate the amount of decline that is clinically significant (i.e., greater than that typically associated with aging at that point in the life span). With age-related changes in sensory capabilities, speed of cognition and response, and perhaps motivation it is also possible that what a task measures for younger adults is different from what it measures for older adults. If test stimuli are very small or require fine hearing discrimination, the performance of older adults could be affected by sensory impairments that

prevent them from seeing or hearing the stimuli.[59–64] What the scale is actually measuring at repeated assessments over a life span could change, for example, from a test
of memory or reasoning to one of vision or hearing. Many older adults with ID in the
current generation were not expected to wear glasses to improve vision or hearing aids
to improve hearing. They often refuse to wear such aids. Thus, it is important to examine
whether a test consistently measures the same thing across persons with differing ages
and abilities. Factors to consider are task demands and changes in functioning that
could affect the ability to meet them (e.g., fine motor skills, slowing with age, etc.).
Such issues are not restricted to direct assessments for dementia. Informants asked to
report on dressing skills, for example, may not mention that adults no longer dress
themselves because arthritis prevents the use of their hands for buttoning, zipping,
pulling, etc. An informant reporting on memory skills may not know that the adult no
longer remembers events seen on television, because they can no longer see or hear
well enough to do so. Thus, it is also important to include vision and hearing screening
as part of any dementia assessment battery.[3,8,10,65]

Etiology of ID

Regarding etiology of ID, individual differences in premorbid strengths and weaknesses
profiles need to be taken into consideration in dementia assessment. Adults with DS
compared to their peers without DS, for example, had a great deal of difficulty placing
small, grooved pegs into a pegboard. They did not place enough pegs into the board
when young and healthy to establish a high enough baseline for further detection of
declines related to dementia. Therefore, a pegboard task involving pegs that were more
easily placed was adopted for dementia assessment, which made it appropriate for
adults with and without DS. Tasks that require clear speech (e.g., picture description,
category fluency) are often difficult to administer to adults who have severe articulation
disorders, because the Examiner cannot understand words clearly enough to know if
they should be scored as correct or not. Often times, such articulation disorders are more
common for adults with DS. Thus, etiology of ID has implications for task appropriate-
ness, as well as cutoff scores for dementia. Such differences need to be taken into
account both at a single assessment and in identifying the amount of change that is
typical over time. Effects of etiology of ID can also interact with other characteristics
(e.g., age, gender) so such interactive effects may also be considered.[66]

Gender

Gender differences have been obtained on a number of tests.[3,8,66,67] It has been
suggested that lower performance in older women with ID is related to estrogen status.[67]
Once again, it is important to know what is typical for adults with ID with varying
characteristics so that performance related to dementia can be identified.

Methods to Address Individual Differences

When deciding who a test is appropriate for, both on a general level and on an individual basis, characteristics such as level of functioning, age, etiology of ID, and gender should be taken into account. Researchers and clinicians have used several methods to take such characteristics into account in scale evaluation.

Homogeneous Groups

One method is to examine the use of a scale in a homogeneous group of adults, for example, all adults with DS over the age of 50 years functioning in the mild range of ID. The use of a homogeneous group eliminates some of the variability in performance and the need to consider performance differences related to some individual differences (in this case etiology of ID, age, and level of functioning). One could conclude with greater certainty that any change over time in healthy adults is typical for this population or that relatively low performance at one assessment is less typical and thus more likely to be associated with dementia. There is still the possibility that premorbid differences in performance related to other variables are present and they need to be considered (e.g., sensory capabilities). The weakness of this homogeneous group method is that one would not know whether a scale validated on such a narrow population would be valid in other populations, such as adults without DS or adults with severe to profound ID. Any scale appropriate for adults with mild ID would also need to be feasibly administered in the later stages of dementia if the scale was to be administered repeatedly (e.g., to examine the natural history of dementia). At times, an adult performs tasks when healthy, but can no longer perform them when demented (i.e., becomes untestable on the test). In such cases, it can be difficult to differentiate "untestable" status related to dementia from that related to other conditions (e.g., depression). Untestable status can also be due to refusal to respond or to loss of the required response because of some other condition (e.g., speech, pointing response). It is best, therefore, to have a test or scale with a range of performance that can detect declines or changes related to dementia.

Stratified Sample

A second strategy for handling individual differences in performance in dementia assessment is to include a heterogeneous, stratified group of adults (e.g., adults with DS ranging from the mild to profound range of functioning). Examiners evaluate performance differences related to individual characteristics and adjustments to cutoff scores, dementia identification rules, or analyses are made.[3,8,12,16,27] Depending on the administration schedule for a given test, such adjustments could be needed for dementia cutoff criteria at a single assessment. They could also be needed for detection of clinically significant declines over repeated assessments. Although the stratified sample method seems advantageous, it can be quite cumbersome in practice to examine and adjust for all possible variations related to individual differences. Ideally, performance on a scale for dementia would not be affected by such individual differences, but as discussed previously all scales, even informant report scales, often must take such differences into account when considering dementia cutoff criteria. In evaluating dementia scales for adults with ID, therefore, it is important to determine how individual differences are handled. One needs to know whether different criteria are needed for adults with different characteristics or whether the test developer has demonstrated that the same criteria apply for all adults. One should also know whether the scale covers a wide enough range of abilities to be appropriate for most adults with ID, or if it is only appropriate for adults with certain levels of premorbid functioning.

Informant Report or Direct Assessment of Performance

An important dementia assessment issue is whether to collect information from informants, from individuals with ID themselves, or from both.[2,10,11,38,56,68] A working group on the diagnosis of dementia recommended both informant report and direct assessment for every evaluation.[1,5,6] They recommended informant report of emotional and everyday functioning, because most adults with ID are not able to reliably report on internal states such as emotions. Similarly, they are not able to monitor their own everyday skills to detect changes. Even adults who are able to report on such states may be unable to do so as dementia progresses. Changes in both emotional and everyday functioning are required for dementia diagnostic criteria to be met.[1]

The working group recommended direct assessment of adults with ID to document memory and cognitive declines as required by dementia diagnostic criteria.[1,5,6] When feasible, direct assessment is usually regarded as preferable to informant report because error related to observation and reporting is not introduced into the assessment. When both informant report and direct assessment are used, consistent information obtained across the two sources is strong support for findings regarding dementia status. Inconsistent information suggests the need for further evaluation or reassessment in the near future.

Informant Report

An important issue in informant reporting is whether the report accurately reflects the functioning of the individual.[2,69] Bias can be introduced if informants find it emotionally difficult to report declines in functioning or depressive signs. Informants may believe that certain declines are not relevant to the person's care and thus may not take note or report them. If an Examiner asks informants to report on unobservable states (e.g., hopelessness), they are required to make an inference about internal states, which may or may not be accurate. Informant report scales on which informants' reports were compared to actual performance would be ideal. The ability of informants to report on the orientation of adults with ID (e.g., knowledge about their name, their place of residence, time) on the DMR,[36] for example, was found to be fair to good.[69] For some orientation items, however, nonverbal IQ, etiology of ID, and age affected level of agreement between informant report and direct performance.

One major obstacle to the use of informant reports of functioning is the availability of consistent, knowledgeable, and reliable informants. Direct care staff often have a high rate of turnover and many adults with ID have older parents who do not live long enough to report on their functioning when they become elderly themselves. Some informant report dementia scales and psychopathology scales require that informants know the individual for 6 months or longer.[2,8,12,70] The informant must also work closely enough with the individual to determine and report on functioning in the last 6 months to a year.[2]

Training has been successfully provided to informants to improve their ability to observe and report on behaviors and functioning relevant to dementia diagnosis.[2] Although not necessary for the use of informant reporting scales, such training would be expected to improve the accuracy and sensitivity of dementia diagnosis. In addition, reliable informant reporting depends on documentation of functioning in the adult's chart and on adequate levels of interrater reliability. Scales requiring reports on current functioning (i.e., in the 2 weeks prior to assessment) are preferable to those requiring retrospective reporting, both because of changes in care providers and because of inaccuracies in informant memory regarding past functioning. If possible, it is ideal for the informant to indicate whether any performance consistent with a dementia diagnosis has always been typical of the individual or not (e.g., adult never knew address of living facility).[2,3,8]

The level of professional expertise required to complete, administer, and interpret informant report scales is another issue to consider. Lay people, such as direct care staff or family members, can complete some scales.[3,69,40,56,70] Highly trained professionals must complete or administer others (e.g., DSDS,[35] most adaptive behavior scales). Some scales require two informants for clinical assessment (e.g., Reiss Screen, DSDS(35)), whereas others rely on one informant (i.e., DMR[36]). Regardless of administration procedures, most dementia diagnostic scales are interpreted by highly trained professionals. There are some scales, however, designed specifically to gather information on a regular basis that is then reported to a diagnostician.[3]

Direct Assessment

Advocates of the sole use of informant report scales often argue that direct tests of individuals with ID for dementia are not feasible or sensitive enough.[71] It has been suggested that adults whose premorbid level of functioning is at or below a mental age of 2 years are often unable to perform neuropsychological tests at a level that would allow detection of declines related to dementia.[3,8] In the experience of members of the working group on dementia assessment, however, most adults with ID can be assessed reliably on direct measures of memory and cognition.[2,3,8,14,16,33,41,68,72,73] Direct assessment has been particularly useful when adults present with signs of both possible dementia and a psychiatric disorder.[52,74] In one instance, for example, informants reported declines in daily functioning and signs of a psychiatric disorder. Direct testing over several years indicated consistent levels of memory and other cognitive functioning, with no apparent declines. Thus, in this case, test performance along with informant data indicated the presence of a potentially treatable psychiatric disorder rather than a progressive, irreversible dementia.[74] As mentioned previously, for any given test there may be individuals who cannot perform its tasks at a clinically useful level (i.e., one that would allow detection of declines), either because of low premorbid functioning or impaired sensory or motor capabilities. The fact that a test does not have universal applicability, however, does not necessarily mean that it is not useful for most adults with ID.

Some care providers report the use of videotaping to directly document changes in functioning related to dementia. Videotaping methods have been used to film assessments for purposes of supervision (i.e., checking on standardized procedures for test administration). Recently videotape recording and data transcription were used to evaluate behavioral excesses (i.e., maladaptive behavior) in adults with dementia.[65] This observational method has the potential to document changes related to dementia, and could be particularly useful for lower functioning individuals or for those with sensory impairments that prevent standard assessments. The challenge would be in developing a method to efficiently provide reliable repeated assessments and clinically useful data.

When directly evaluating adults with ID for dementia, it is important to follow best assessment practices.[75] Qualified evaluators should conduct the assessment, particularly those who have experience working with individuals with ID. Untrained Examiners sometimes have biased notions about the abilities of people with ID. They may not expect them to perform tasks they are perfectly capable of completing, thus biasing results. Testing should be conducted in a room free of distractions. When selecting and interpreting the results from specific tests or scales, the characteristics of the individual should be considered (e.g., lack of speech, apparent level of motivation, etc.). Most adults with ID enjoy the one-on-one attention typical of a testing experience and benefit from reinforcement of effort. Further considerations specific for dementia assessment are time of day, given that the course of dementia varies across the day with optimal functioning often in the morning.

A question remains as to whether the sole use of either informant report or direct assessment measures is sufficient to make a diagnosis of dementia or to document declines in functioning. Batteries involving both informant report and direct assessment measures led to higher levels of sensitivity and specificity than informant report alone.[3,8,16] Direct assessment was used to assess memory and cognitive functioning, whereas informant report was used to assess emotional and everyday functioning.

Source of information was confounded, therefore, with which diagnostic criteria were being assessed. The relative contribution of informant report versus direct assessment in the diagnosis of dementia in adults with ID, therefore, is an issue that requires further examination. It is possible that their respective values could vary with the characteristics of individuals being assessed.[11]

Evaluation of Assessment Scales and Techniques

When examining dementia assessment scales and diagnostic techniques, it is necessary to determine how the scale or technique was evaluated. Evaluation usually involves comparisons of dementia status as determined by using the scale to that determined by an independent source. These comparisons involve an examination of scale sensitivity, specificity, predictive validity, test–retest reliability, and clinical usefulness.[2,3,8,12,17,41,43] Ideally, all of these measures would be optimized for any given scale or technique. A validation technique that is sometimes used involves group comparisons, so they are also discussed here. The role of dementia stage in the assessment process is also considered.

Independent/External Validation Criterion

To determine whether test performance or behavior reported by an informant are valid indicators of dementia, one must have an independent way to document whether individuals are demented or not. If the scale differentiates those who are demented from those who are not, then there is support for its use. Unfortunately, there are no biological indicators for use as a gold standard for dementia.[13,76] Historically, diagnosis of dementia by an experienced clinician was used as a gold standard. There is evidence, however, that some clinicians are biased to diagnose more dementia in adults with DS than adults with other forms of ID.[3,8,47] An alternative validation method is to combine clinician diagnosis with diagnosis based on objective test results to arrive at a consensus diagnosis of dementia.[2,16,20] This method has less potential for bias, particularly if the clinician is blind to the age of the adult or to the etiology of ID.[2,4] Still others have confirmed the presence of DAD by requiring that all adults so diagnosed show declines in functioning for 2–3 consecutive years.[12] Finally, investigators have used previously developed scales with demonstrated validity to examine the validity of new methods.[2,3,7,15,16,20,72] Thus, the demonstrated validity of the new scale depends on the validity of the existing scale. Although there is currently no ideal solution for the selection of external validation criteria for dementia scales, it is important to remember that the choice of external validation criteria can have repercussions for obtained sensitivity and specificity of tests (i.e., the extent to which a test correctly identifies those who are demented and those who are not demented, respectively).

Sensitivity, Specificity, and Predictive Value

As illustrated in Table 2.2, cutoff rules are often used to indicate whether a given individual has declines in functioning consistent with dementia.[2,3,8,12,17,41,43] On a single test, adults with scores above a certain cutoff, for example, would be considered demented, whereas those with scores below the cutoff would be considered not demented. As seen in Table 2.2, one could set the cutoff rules liberally (i.e., a lower cutoff score) so that more adults are identified as demented. More conservative cutoff rules (i.e., higher cutoff score) would mean that fewer adults are identified as demented.[2,3,8] If a test battery is used, liberal cutoff rules could involve documentation of declines needed to meet any two diagnostic criteria (e.g., memory and everyday functioning). More conservative rules, in contrast, could require declines or changes such that all diagnostic criteria are met (memory, cognitive, everyday, and emotional

Table 2.2 Effect of Different Cutoff Rules on Dementia Scale Evaluation Measures[a]

Dementia Classifications based on Scale Cutoff Rules and External Criterion

Liberal cutoff rule on scale	External criterion		Conservative cutoff rule on scale	External criterion	
	Demented	Not demented		Demented	Not demented
Demented	63	20	Demented	58	2
Not demented	7	10	Not demented	12	28

Evaluation measures by cutoff rule

Measure	Liberal rule	Conservative rule
Sensitivity	.90	.83
Specificity	.33	.93
Positive predictive value	.76	.97
Negative predictive value	.59	.70

Note: Sensitivity refers to a scale's ability to correctly identify adults considered to be demented (i.e., 63/70 and 58/70 for liberal and conservative cutoff rules, respectively). Specificity refers to a scale's ability to correctly identify adults considered to be not demented (i.e., 10/30 and 28/30 for liberal and conservative cutoff rules, respectively). Positive and negative predictive values refer to whether demented and not demented adults identified by the scale receive matching diagnoses from an external criterion (e.g., positive predictive value for liberal data is 63/83).

[a]Data were created to demonstrate differences in evaluation measures for liberal versus conservative cutoff rules. Liberal rules applied to one scale, for example, would require a lower cutoff score as an indication of dementia compared to a more conservative higher cutoff score (with higher scores indicating more severe dementia symptoms). Liberal rules applied to a battery of tests could require that only two diagnostic criteria are met (e.g., declines in memory and everyday functioning), whereas a conservative rule could require that all diagnostic criteria are met (i.e., memory and other cognitive declines, emotional changes, declines in everyday functioning).

functioning).[2,3,8,16] Adults would be classified based on the cutoff rules as demented or not demented (although classifications of possible dementia are also useful). The dementia classifications based on the rules are then compared to those based on an external criterion (e.g., clinical judgment, existing dementia scale classifications). Scale evaluation measures are then calculated as described in the note to Table 2.2.

As indicated by the example, the use of a more liberal cutoff rule may increase the sensitivity of a scale at the cost of specificity. That is, more adults would be identified as demented. Some of them, however, would not be demented according to the external comparison criterion. Similarly, the use of a more conservative cutoff rule could increase specificity at the cost of sensitivity. In this case, fewer adults are identified as demented, but some of them are considered to be demented according to the external criterion. At times, one may want a scale or technique to be more sensitive, such as when using it as a general screen for dementia or other psychiatric disorders. At other times, one would want a scale or technique to be more specific, such as when telling family members that an adult with ID has an irreversible dementia, as opposed to some potentially treatable psychiatric disorder. When using evaluation measures such as those illustrated in Table 2.2, one must consider issues discussed previously. Did the scale and external criterion, for example, use the same source of information when evaluating dementia? If the scale was a direct assessment scale like a memory test or battery of tests and the criterion was an informant report scale like a dementia scale, lack of agreement could occur simply because of the different sources of information. Of course, if a scale is useful, one would expect it to agree diagnostically with other valid scales designed for the same population (e.g., adults with DS with mild ID) regardless of the source of information.[2,69] When examining predictive validity, one could determine whether dementia status on the scale agrees with that determined by the external criterion at one point in time. One could also determine whether dementia status or declines in functioning on the scale at time 1 predict dementia status according to the external criterion at time 2 several years later.[2,3,8]

Reliability

A dementia assessment method that is to be used repeatedly must have adequate test–retest reliability. One way to examine such reliability is simply to repeat the assessment in healthy adults to see if the scores or dementia classifications remain the same. If informant report techniques are used, the same informant would need to report on functioning at each assessment, which can sometimes be challenging because of turnover in direct care staff. When using direct assessment techniques, practice effects can affect repeated test performance even when tests are administered after a long time interval.[3,8] Changes in test performance that could be related to aging as opposed to dementia should also be considered when evaluating test–retest reliability. Another way to examine test–retest reliability and perhaps the validity of a more complex test is to see whether the underlying factor structure remains the same over time. For example, an informant-report dementia scale could involve assessment of depression, memory, and maladaptive behavior. Items believed to assess these three areas should have a consistent factor structure over time if they are actually measuring the same thing.[3]

Finally, informant-report scales given at a single assessment or repeatedly should have adequate interrater reliability. Some informant-report scales require the use of two informants and thus allow examination of interrater agreement at each assessment (e.g., DSDS[35]; Reiss Screen[70]). If a scale requiring just one rater has demonstrated interrater reliability, then changes in informants from one assessment to the next would not be expected to result in drastic changes in reported performance, like those expected with dementia. If an adult has reported declines in performance and the informant has changed, however, it can be difficult to conclude that actual declines have taken place. Sometimes, a change in informant coincides with a change to a more restrictive or assistive living environment. If this is the case, it is difficult to separate changes in reported behavior due to informant perceptions from those due to changes in the environment.

Group Comparisons

At times dementia scales or diagnostic techniques are evaluated by comparing the performance of groups with and without dementia. A memory test is administered to adults with and without dementia, for example, and performance is compared. If the adults with dementia score lower than those without dementia, however, several issues must be addressed when interpreting such findings. First, there is the issue of confounding factors affecting performance that could differ between the groups (e.g., level of functioning, age, etiology of ID, medical health, sensory capabilities, etc.). Second, one must interpret overlapping performance between the groups (i.e., individual adults in both the demented and not demented group could remember five items). It is possible that an adult with dementia remembered 8–10 items when healthy, but declined to the current level. The adult without dementia, in contrast, could be showing optimal performance. Without an indication of performance for the individuals in the demented group when healthy, one does not necessarily know that the memory test would actually differentiate those with dementia from those without. In some cases the test being evaluated is initially used to determine whether adults are demented or not (e.g., an adult with a score of 5 or lower on the memory test is demented, otherwise they are not). In such cases, group assignment is not independent of the evaluation of the scale, and reliable conclusions about the scales' usefulness cannot be made.

Evaluation and Stages of Dementia

When evaluating dementia scales and techniques, the value of the results could vary as a function of the stage of dementia (given a progressive dementia).[9] Some adults when healthy, for example, function independently in the community with a large array of academic and vocational skills. If they decline to the more advanced stages of dementia and need full time care, few individuals would argue over the presence of clinically significant declines. In such instances, high agreement would be expected among different dementia diagnostic methods. At earlier stages of dementia, however, the individual may show some behavioral changes (e.g., uncharacteristically telling stories about what they have done or what others will do). In such instances, it is often unclear whether clinically significant declines in functioning as required by diagnostic criteria have occurred (i.e., declines in memory, other cognitive, emotional, and everyday functioning). If a psychiatric disorder is present (e.g., depression), it is also difficult to determine the extent to which losses in functioning are related to the disorder versus an underlying dementia.[7,52,74] One must determine whether a psychiatric disorder such as depression or a psychosis could lead to such a change in functioning. It is at this stage of dementia, specifically with psychiatric symptoms complicating diagnostic issues, when agreement among different dementia diagnostic methods would be expected to be lower. It is at this stage, however, when dementia scales could be most beneficial, because treatment could be most beneficial.[77-83] Future research will be needed to determine the clinical usefulness of classifications like "possible dementia" or "preclinical dementia" which are used in the general population when dementia is suspected but definitely confirmed. Scales and techniques allowing such classifications, however, would be advantageous at this point.[3,7,8,41]

Stage of dementia could also affect the obtained sensitivity of dementia scales. It can be very difficult for care providers and family members to detect early signs of dementia (particularly those in memory and cognition). Therefore, an adult who has already shown undetected declines in functioning could be referred for screening. As such, the declines usually detected by a given scale used for screening or evaluation could never be detected because they occurred before the adult came to the attention of clinicians or researchers. A number of researchers and clinicians have addressed this issue by identifying and assessing only adults when they change from a healthy to a demented status. This is the ideal method for examining the sensitivity and predictive value of a scale. It is often not practical, however, because of the need to include in analyses all adults identified with dementia at a given site, because of small numbers detected with dementia. In addition, clinicians do not always have the luxury of having a baseline record of healthy functioning, and they must make diagnostic decisions based on the stage of dementia present when the adult is first evaluated. Therefore, it would be beneficial when evaluating scales to determine their validity as a function of the stage of dementia.

Evaluation and Strength/Weakness Profile

Evaluation results could also be affected by premorbid level of functioning and profile of strengths and weaknesses. If, for example, adults with milder levels of ID typically scored at the ceiling of a test, the test may not be able to differentiate those who have started to show declines in functioning from others until they are in the more advanced stages. The test, however, could be an excellent indicator of dementia in lower functioning individuals. Similarly, if a test is so difficult or the instructions are so complex that healthy, lower functioning adults score at the floor of the test or at a level that would not allow detection of declines, then the test would not be a good indicator of dementia for them. It could, however, be an excellent indicator of dementia for higher functioning adults, whose functioning on such a test could be highly indicative of dementia status. Similarly, adults with a premorbid weakness in an area (e.g., due to sensory impairments or articulation disorders) could affect test evaluation results in unexpected ways. Thus, when evaluating a test it is important to consider individual differences related to level of functioning, age, gender, and etiology of ID as discussed previously. At this time, it is not known whether one test or set of tests or scales is useful for adults at all levels of functioning. It is possible that tests or scales specific to level of functioning could lead to maximal levels of sensitivity and specificity, at least for adults with milder levels of ID.

Clinical Usefulness of Dementia Assessment Scales and Techniques

A final issue in scale evaluation is whether the scale would actually be useful and feasible to administer in a clinical setting. Often scales and techniques are evaluated as part of a research project, and the usefulness of the scale or technique has not been evaluated in a clinical setting. Questions shown in Appendix 1 address the issue of clinical usefulness.

Summary

What can seem like a staggering number of issues affects the assessment of dementia in adults with ID. Such issues, however, are similar to those pertinent to the assessment of dementia in the general population for whom a considerable amount of effort and resources has been devoted.[84] Extra effort, such as that demonstrated by the authors of subsequent chapters, is required for scale development and evaluation for adults with ID. Each chapter will discuss a number of issues related to their respective tests or scales.

References

1. Aylward EH, Burt DB, Thorpe LU et al. (1997) Diagnosis of dementia in individuals with intellectual disability. J Intellect Disabil Res 41: 152–164.

2. Ball SL, Holland AJ, Huppert FA et al. (2004) The modified CAMDEX informant interview is a valid and reliable tool for use in the diagnosis of dementia in adults with Down's syndrome. J Intellect Disabil Res 48: 611–620.

3. Burt DB, Primeaux-Hart S, Loveland KA et al. (2005) Comparing dementia diagnostic methods used with people with intellectual disabilities. J Policy Pract Intellect Disabil 2: 94–115.

4. Holland AJ, Hon J, Huppert FA et al. (2000) Incidence and course of dementia in people with Down's syndrome: Findings from a population-based study. J Intellect Disabil Res 44: 138–146.

5. Burt DB and Aylward E. (2000) Test battery for the diagnosis of dementia in individuals with intellectual disability. J Intellect Disabil Res 44: 175–180.

6. Burt DB and Aylward E. (1998) Test Battery for the Diagnosis of Dementia in Individuals with Intellectual Disability. Washington: American Association on Mental Retardation.

7. Ball SL, Holland AJ, Hon J et al. (2006). Personality and behaviour changes mark the early stages of Alzheimer's disease in adults with Down's syndrome: findings from a prospective population-based study. Int J Geriatr Psychiatry. 21:661-673.

8. Burt DB, Primeaux-Hart S, Loveland KA et al. (2005) Tests and medical conditions associated with dementia diagnosis. J Policy Pract Intellect Disabil 2: 47–56.

9. Devenny DA, Krinsky-McHale SJ, Sersen G et al. (2000) Sequence of cognitive decline in dementia in adults with Down's syndrome. J Intellect Disabil Res 44: 654–665.

10. Kalsy S, McQuillan S, Adams D et al. (2005) A proactive psychological screening strategy for dementia in adults with Down syndrome: Preliminary description of service use and evaluation. J Policy Pract Intellect Disabil 2: 116–125.

11. Kay DW, Tyrer SP, Margallo-Lana ML et al. (2003) Preliminary evaluation of a scale to assess cognitive function in adults with Down syndrome: The Prudhoe Cognitive Function Test. J Intellect Disabil Res 47: 155–168.

12. Prasher VP. (1997) Dementia Questionnaire for Persons with Mental Retardation (DMR). Modified criteria for adults with Down's syndrome. J Appl Res Intellect Disabil 10: 54–60.

13. Prasher VP. (2006) Macrocytosis: a peripheral marker for dementia in Alzheimer's disease in adults with Down syndrome ? In Prasher V, editor. Down Syndrome and Alzheimer's Disease, Biological Correlates. Oxon, UK: Radcliffe Publishing.

14. Sano M, Aisen PS, Dalton AJ et al. (2005) Assessment of aging individuals with Down syndrome in clinical trials: Results of baseline measures. J Policy Pract Intellect Disabil 2: 126–138.

15. Shultz J, Aman M, Kelbl ey T et al. (2004) Evaluation of screening tools for dementia in older adults with mental retardation. Am J Ment Retard 109: 98–110.

16. Silverman W, Schupf N, Zigman W et al. (2004) Dementia in adults with mental retardation: Assessment at a single point in time. Am J Ment Retard 109: 111–125.

17. Palmer GA. (2006) Neuropsychological profiles of persons with mental retardation and dementia. Res Dev Disabil 27: 299–308.

18. Visser FE, Aldenkamp AP, van Huffelen AC et al. (1997) Prospective study of the prevalence of Alzheimer-type dementia in institutionalized individuals with Down syndrome. Am J Ment Retard 101: 400–412.

19. Nelson LD, Orme D, Osann K et al. (2001) Neurological changes and emotional functioning in adults with Down Syndrome. J Intellect Disabil Res 45: 450–456.

20. Zigman WB, Schupf N, Devenny DA et al. (2004) Incidence and prevalence of dementia in elderly adults with mental retardation without Down syndrome. Am J Ment Retard 109: 126–141.

21. Burt DB, Primeaux-Hart S, Loveland KA et al. (2005) Aging in adults with intellectual disabilities. Am J Ment Retard 110: 268–284.

22. Busch A and Beail N. (2004) Risk factors for dementia in people with Down syndrome: Issues in assessment and diagnosis. Am J Ment Retard 109: 83–97.

23. Holland AJ, Hon J, Huppert F et al. (1998) Population-based study of the prevalence and presentation of dementia in adults with Down's syndrome. Br J Psychiatry 172: 493–498.

24. Burt DB and Aylward EH. (1999) Assessment methods for diagnosis of dementia. In: Janicki M and Dalton A, editors. Dementia, Aging, and Intellectual Disabilities: A Handbook. Philadelphia, PA: Taylor & Francis.

25. Dalton AJ and Crapper-McLachlan DR. (1984) Incidence of memory deterioration in aging persons with Down's syndrome. In: Berg JM, editor. Perspectives and Progress in Mental Retardation, Vol. 2. Biomedical Aspects. Austin, TX: PRO-ED.

26. Hewitt KE, Carter G and Jancar J. (1985) Ageing in Down's syndrome. Br J Psychiatry 147: 58–62.

27. Evenhuis HM. (1990) The natural history of dementia in Down's syndrome. Arch Neurol 47: 263–267.

28. Lai F and Williams RS. (1989) A prospective study of Alzheimer disease in Down syndrome. Arch Neurol 46: 849–853.

29. Gedye A. (1998) Neuroleptic-induced dementia documented in four adults with mental retardation. Ment Retard 36: 182–186.

30. Burt DB. (1999) Dementia and depression. In: Janicki M and Dalton A, editors. Dementia, Aging, and Intellectual Disabilities: A Handbook. Philadelphia, PA: Taylor & Francis.

31. Thorpe LU. (1999) Psychiatric disorders. In: Janicki M and Dalton A, editors. Dementia, Aging, and Intellectual Disabilities: A Handbook. Philadelphia, PA: Taylor & Francis.

32. Tsiouris JA. (1999) Psychotropic medications. In: Janicki M and Dalton A, editors. Dementia, Aging, and Intellectual Disabilities: A Handbook. Philadelphia, PA: Taylor & Francis.

33. Dalton AJ and Fedor BL. (1998) Onset of dyspraxia in aging persons with Down syndrome: Longitudinal studies. J Intellect Dev Disabil 23: 13–24.

34. Folstein MF, Folstein SE, and McHugh PR. (1975) Mini-Mental State: A practical method for grading the cognitive state of patients for the clinician. J Psychiatry Res 12: 189–198.

35. Gedye A. (1985) Dementia Scale for Down syndrome. Manual. Vancouver, BC: Gedye Research and Consulting.

36. Evenhuis HM, Kengen MMF, and Eurlings HAL. (1990) Dementia Questionnaire for Mentally Retarded Persons. Zwannerdam, the Netherlands: Hooge Burch Institute for Mentally Retarded People.

37. Janicki M and Dalton A, editors. (1999) Dementia, Aging, and Intellectual Disabilities: A Handbook. Philadelphia, PA: Taylor & Francis.

38. Strydom A and Hassiotis A. (2003) Diagnostic instruments for dementia in older people with intellectual disability in clinical practice. Aging Mental Health 7: 432–437.

39. Evenhuis HM, Kengen MMF, and Eurlings HA. (1998) Dementie Vragenlijst voor Verstandelijk Gehandicapten (DVZ). Tweede, geheel gewijzigde druk, Harcourt Test Publishers, Amsterdam.

40. Evenhuis HM, Kengen MMF, and Eurlings HAL. (2006) Dementia Questionnaire for Persons with Intellectual Disabilities (DMR). Amsterdam: Harcourt Test Publishers.

41. Devenny DA, Zimmerli EJ, Kittle P et al. (2002) Cued recall in early-stage dementia in adults with Down's syndrome. J Intellect Disabil Res 46: 472–483.

42. Kittler P, Krinsky-McHale SJ, and Devenny DA. (2006) Verbal intrusions precede memory decline in adults with Down syndrome. J Intellect Disabil Res 50: 1–10.

43. Krinsky-McHale SJ, Devenny DA, and Silverman WP. (2002) Changes in explicit memory associated with early dementia in adults with Down's syndrome. J Intellect Disabil Res 46: 198–208.

44. Krinsky-McHale SJ, Devenny DA, Kittler PK et al. (2006) Assessing selective attention deficits in adults with DS and DAT. In: Paper Presented at the 38th Annual Gatlinburg Conference on Research and Theory in Mental Retardation and Developmental Disabilities, Annapolis, MD.

45. Prasher V, Farooq A, and Holder R. (2004) The Adaptive Behaviour Questionnaire (ABDQ): Screening questionnaire for dementia in Alzheimer's disease in adults with Down syndrome. Res Dev Disabil 25: 385–397.

46. Urv TK, Zigman WB, and Silverman W. (2003) Maladaptive behaviors related to adaptive decline in aging adults with mental retardation. Am J Ment Retard 108: 327–339.

47. Acquilano JP. (2006) Differential diagnosis of Alzheimer's disease. Unpublished doctoral dissertation. Capella University, Minneapolis, MN.
48. Acquilano JP, Davidson PW, Henderson CM et al. (2003) Functional skills and health status in older persons with intellectual disabilities. In: Paper Presented at the13th Annual Roundtable of the International Association for the Scientific Study of Intellectual Disabilities, Volos, Greece.
49. Chicoine B, McGuire D, Hebein S et al. (1994) Development of a clinic for adults with Down syndrome. Ment Retard 32: 100–106.
50. Chicoine B, McGuire D, and Rubin S. (1999) Specialty clinic perspectives. In: Janicki MP and Dalton AJ, editors. Dementia, Aging, and Intellectual Disabilities: A Handbook. Philadelphia, PA: Brunner/Mazel.
51. Davidson PW, Janicki MP, Ladrigan P et al. (2003) Associations between behavior disorders and health status among older adults with intellectual disability. Aging Mental Health 7: 424–430.
52. Devenny DA, Wegiel J, Schupf N et al (2005) Dementia of the Alzheimer's type and accelerated aging in Down syndrome. Science. SAGE KE. http://sageke.sciencemag.org/cgi/content/full/2005/14/dn1.
53. Henderson CM and Davidson PW. (2000) Comprehensive adult and geriatric assessment. In: Janicki MP and Ansello EF, editors. Community Supports for Aging Adults with Lifelong Disabilities. Baltimore, MD: Paul H. Brookes.
54. Holland AJ. (1999) Psychiatry and mental retardation. Int Rev Psychiatry 11: 76–82.
55. Patti PJ, Amble KB, and Flory MJ. (2005) Life events in older adults with intellectual disabilities: Differences between adults with and without Down syndrome. J Policy Pract Intellect Disabil 2: 149–155.
56. Prosser H, Moss S, Costello H et al (1998) Reliability and validity of the Mini PAS-ADD for assessing psychiatric disorders in adults with intellectual disability. J Intellect Disabil Res. 42: 264–272.
57. Van Schrojenstein Lantman-deValk, HMJ, van den Akker M, Maskaant MA et al. (1997) Prevalence and incidence of health problems in people with intellectual disability. J Intellect Disabil Res 41: 42–51.
58. Hawkins BA, Eklund SJ, James DR et al. (2003) Adaptive behavior and cognitive function of adults with Down syndrome: Modeling change with age. Ment Retard 41: 7–28.
59. Castane M, Boada-Rovira M, and Hernandez-Ruia I. (2004) Eye conditions as features of Down's syndrome in patients over 40 years of age. Rev Neurol 39: 1017–1021.
60. Evenhuis HM. (1995) Medical aspects of ageing in a population with intellectual disability: I. Visual impairment. J Intellect Disabil Res 39: 19–25.
61. Evenhuis HM. (1995) Medical aspects of ageing in a population with intellectual disability: II. Hearing impairment. J Intellect Disabil Res 39: 27–33.
62. Fisher K and Kettl P. (2005) Aging with mental retardation: increasing population of older adults with MR require health interventions and prevention strategies. Geriatrics 60: 26–29.
63. Krinsky-McHale SJ, Abramov I, Devenny DA et al. (2001) Visual deficits in adults with Down syndrome. In: Paper Presented at the 34th annual Gatlinburg Conference on Research and Theory in Mental Retardation and Developmental Disabilities, Charleston, SC.
64. Woodhouse JM, Adler P, and Duignan A (2004) Vision in athletes with intellectual disabilities: The need for improved eyecare. J Intellect Disabil Res 48: 736–745.
65. Millichap D, Oliver C, McQuillan S et al. (2003) Descriptive functional analysis of behavioral excesses shown by adults with Down syndrome and dementia. Int J Geriatr Psychiatry 18: 844–854.
66. Kittler P, Krinsky-McHale SJ, and Devenny DA. (2004) Sex differences in performance over 7 years on the Wechsler Intelligence Scale for Children—Revised among adults with intellectual disability. J Intellect Disabil Res 48: 114–122.
67. Schupf N, Pang D, Patel BN et al. (2003) Onset of dementia is associated with age at menopause in women with Down's syndrome. Ann Neurol 54: 433–438.

68. Oliver, C (1999) Perspectives on assessment and evaluation. In: Janicki M and Dalton A, editors. Dementia, Aging, and Intellectual Disabilities: A Handbook. Philadelphia, PA: Taylor & Francis.
69. Burt DB, Primeaux-Hart S, Phillips NB et al. (1999) Assessment of orientation: Relationship between informant report and direct measures. Ment Retard. 37: 364–370.
70. Reiss S. (1986) Manual for the Reiss Screen for Maladaptive Behavior: Version 1.1. New York: International Diagnostic Systems.
71. Deb S and Braganza J. (1999) Comparison of rating scales for the diagnosis of dementia in adults with Down's syndrome. J Intellect Disabil Res 43: 400–407.
72. Oliver C, Holland A, Hall S et al. (2005) The assessment of memory impairment in adults with Down syndrome: The effect of increasing task load on test sensitivity. Am J Ment Retard 110: 339–345.
73. Cosgrave MP, McCarron M, Anderson M et al. (1998) Cognitive decline in Down syndrome: A validity/reliability study of the Test for Severe Impairment. Am J Ment Retard 103: 193–197.
74. Burt DB, Loveland KA, Primeaux-Hart S et al. (1998) Dementia in adults with Down syndrome: Diagnostic challenges. Am J Ment Retard. 103: 130–145.
75. Aylward EH, Burt DB, Thorpe Lu et al. (1995) Diagnosis of Dementia in Individuals with Intellectual Disability. Washington, DC: American Association of Mental Retardation.
76. Prasher V, Cumella S, Natarajan K et al. (2003) Magnetic resonance imaging, Down's syndrome and Alzheimer's disease: Research and clinical implications. J Intellect Disabil Res 47: 90–100.
77. Boada-Rovira M, Hernandez-Ruiz I, Badenas-Homiar S et al. (2005) Clinical-therapeutic study of dementia in people with Down syndrome and the effectiveness of donepezil in this population. Rev Neurol 41: 129–136.
78. Cipriani G, Bianchetti A, and Travucchi M. (2003) Donepezil use in the treatment of dementia associated with Down syndrome. Arch Neurol 60: 292.
79. Lott IT, Osann K, Doran E et al. (2002) Down syndrome and Alzheimer disease: Response to donepezil. Arch Neurol 59: 1133–1136.
80. Prasher VP. (2004) Review of donepezil, rivastigmine, galantamine and memantine for the treatment of dementia in Alzheimer's disease in adults with Down syndrome: Implications for the intellectual disability population. Int J Geriatr Psychiatry 19: 509–515.
81. Prasher VP, Adams C, and Holder R. (2003) Long term safety and efficacy of donepezil in the treatment of dementia in Alzheimer's disease in adults with Down syndrome: Open label study. Int J Geriatr Psychiatry 18: 549–551.
82. Prasher VP, Fung N, and Adams C. (2005) Rivastigmine in the treatment of dementia in Alzheimer's disease in adults with Down syndrome. Int J Geriatr Psychiatry 20: 496–497.
83. Prasher VP, Huxley A, Haque MS et al. (2002) A 24-week, double-blind, placebo-controlled trial of donepezil in patients with Down syndrome and Alzheimer's disease—Pilot study. Int J Geriatr Psychiatry 17: 270–278.
84. Small GW, Rabins PV, Barry PP et al. (1997) Diagnosis and treatment of Alzheimer disease and related disorders. Consensus statement of the American Association for Geriatric Psychiatry, the Alzheimer's Association, and the American Geriatrics Society. J Am Med Assoc 278: 1363–71.

Chapter 3
The Dementia Questionnaire for People with Intellectual Disabilities

H.M. Evenhuis, M.M.F. Kengen, and H.A.L. Eurlings

Introduction

To facilitate the diagnosis of dementia in persons with intellectual disabilities (ID), based on observations of caregivers, since 1980 the Dementie Vragenlijst voor Zwakzinnigen (DVZ) has been developed by Heleen Evenhuis, ID physician, and Margeen Kengen and Harry Eurlings, behavioral therapists, all working in De Bruggen center for people with ID, Zwammerdam, the Netherlands.[1] The Dementia Questionnaire for People with Intellectual Disabilities (DMR) is an English translation of this instrument. After many years of distribution through De Bruggen, its publication has now been taken over by Harcourt Test Publishers.[2] In this chapter, we review the DMR.

Background

In people without a preexisting cognitive impairment, the diagnosis of dementia is primarily based upon an interview with the patient and his/her family. Collected information concerns memory, orientation, thought, mood, interest and activities, self-care, speech, and practical abilities. Completed with neuropsychological assessment, and physical and laboratory assessment to exclude physical causes of deterioration, a diagnosis of probable dementia can be made in an early stage in a vast majority of cases. Our practical experience at that moment, later confirmed by research, was that in principle, dementia has in people with ID the same course and similar symptoms as in other people.[3,4] Therefore, the diagnostic procedure should be comparable. Because neuropsychological tests, at least those available in those years, were not applicable to persons with developmental ages lower than around 5 or 6 years, we considered a careful interview of observations by the family or other carers of even more importance for a diagnosis than in other people. To help us and others ask the right questions, we decided to develop a list of items, which should be normally asked in each proxy-based interview.

V.P. Prasher (ed.), *Neuropsychological Assessments of Dementia in Down Syndrome and Intellectual Disabilities*,
DOI: 10.1007/978-1-84800-249-4_3, © Springer Science+Business Media, LLC 2009

DMR Designing Process

We started with the normal way in patient interviews, designing our item list accordingly: what is the situation now, and what was it before that? Before long we were confronted with the problem, that in this population, the preexisting cognitive level varies considerably between individuals. Therefore, the current functional level will always, more explicitly than in other people, have to be compared with the former level of functioning. This can only be realized in case of continuous and capable observations by persons who are familiar with the individual person and with symptoms of dementia. However, in practice, the average carer worked no longer than 2 years with the same clients, whereas, in the 1980s, nobody had any experience with dementia. Especially memory and orientation were seldom explicitly noted. As a result, observations were always incomplete and relevant data had been unsatisfactorily recorded. We concluded that looking back did not provide us with reliable, objective information, and that we had to work the other way round: structured recording of functioning before any deterioration was apparent, and again in case of deterioration. This required questions in a "here and now" format. Moreover, they had to be formulated in such a way, that they could be answered for persons with mild, moderate as well as severe ID.

These considerations resulted in a first draft with 77 items, to be completed by a family or staff member, who was familiar with the person. The questions were primarily based on first international guidelines for dementia diagnosis,[5,6] and were originally clustered in seven clinical subscales: short-term memory, long-term memory, spatial and temporal orientation, speech, practical skills, mood and inactivity, and behavioral disturbance. Further, the choice of items was based on our practical experience with interests and communicative capacities of people with mild to severe ID. Together with the methodologist Prof. L.J.Th. van der Kamp of the psychology department of Leiden University, and his graduate student Josien de Boer, the format was completed and first evaluation studies were performed. To prevent response tendencies, the items were placed in an arbitrary sequence. The questionnaire was provided with a simple linear score system, in which the items had three response categories: 0 points, no deficit; 1 point, moderate deficit; 2 points, severe deficit. Therefore, higher scores correspond to more severe deterioration. Appendix 2 shows the format of questions 1–5.

The subject's behavior during the past 2 months had to be judged. If an item could not be defined, e.g., in case of a lack of expressive capacities of the subject, this could be scored as "not to be determined" in the early version.

First Studies, Leading to Publication of the Final Version

In 1983, single completions of the first version of the DMR were performed by pairs of two independent carers for 98 institutionalized older persons with mild to profound ID, to test the interrater reliability, internal consistency of the subscales,

Table 3.1 Dementia Questionnaire for People with ID (DMR)

Subscales	Min-max scores
Sum of cognitive scores (SCS)	0–44
1. Short-term memory (seven items)	0–14
2. Long-term memory (eight items)	0–16
3. Spatial and temporal orientation (seven items)	0–14
Sum of social scores (SOS)	0–60
4. Speech (4 items)	0–8
5. Practical skills (8 items)	0–16
6. Mood (6 items)	0–12
7. Activity and interest (6 items)	0–12
8. Behavioral disturbance (6 items)	0–12

and the relationship of intellectual levels and scores. The interrater reliability appeared satisfactory (see below). Items that correlated insufficiently with the other items within the same subscale, were omitted, as well as items that in a majority were scored as "not to be determined" and items which discriminated insufficiently (i.e., mostly scored as "0"), leading to a final list of 50 questions (Table 3.1).

As expected, a negative correlation was found between intellectual levels and scores: the lower the intellectual level, the higher the scores. Based on internal consistency outcomes, the original subscale "Mood and Inactivity" was split up into the subscales "Mood" and "Activity and Interest."[7] In a second study, again with single completions, in two institutionalized populations of, respectively, 271 and 263 older persons with mild to profound ID, the relationship of the expert diagnosis "dementia" with DMR scores was studied. Results of a discriminant analysis showed that the subscales "Short-term memory," "Orientation," "Speech," "Practical skills," and "Mood" discriminated best between groups with and without a diagnosis "dementia." If scores of all individual participants were classified according to the results of the discriminant analysis, in an average of 72% of subjects a correct diagnosis was made. A correct diagnosis based on DMR scores appeared particularly difficult in case of a severe or profound ID, extreme apathy, or clouded consciousness.[8]

Psychometric Properties

Reliability

The interrater reliability was studied by measuring the Pearson correlation coefficient for the different subscales. In this stage of the development of the DMR, the subscales "Mood" and "Activity and interest" were one subscale. The correlation coefficients for the different subscales varied between .44 and .94 (Table 3.2). Only for subscale "Behavioral disturbance," the correlation between raters was relatively low (.44). It appeared that this low correlation resulted from differences within one of the six pairs of raters. The results for the other subscales were satisfactory.[7]

Table 3.2 Interrater Reliability[7]

Subscale	Pearson correlation coefficient
Short-term memory	.84
Long-term memory	.87
Orientation	.86
Speech	.68
Practical skills	.94
Mood/activity and interest	.74
Behavioral disturbance	.44

"Gold Standard": Expert Diagnosis

Because no other diagnostic instruments for dementia were available, evaluated for people with ID, a specialist diagnosis by a physician and/or psychologist with expert knowledge in the field of dementia and ID was used against which to judge the sensitivity of DMR scores. A specialist diagnosis "dementia" was made in case of a permanent and increasing deterioration of the cognitive and social functioning, according to DSM-III-R and later DSM-IV criteria.[5,9] These criteria had to be slightly modified (Table 3.3), because of the variance of original cognitive functioning as part of the ID. Additionally, because no or hardly any neuropsychological test methods are available to reliably assess abstract thought, judgment, aphasia, apraxia or constructive insight in this population, we omitted the criterion "disturbances of abstract thought and judgment," whereas aphasia and apraxia could only be observed in daily circumstances.

Sensitivity and Specificity

In two prospective longitudinal studies, the sensitivity and specificity of different criteria for interpretation of DMR scores have been studied in older groups with Down syndrome (DS) and with other causes of ID, both for multiple and for single completions.[10,11] In these studies, persons with a clinical expert diagnosis of "dubious dementia" were classified as demented. The diagnosis "dubious dementia" was made in all cases of progressive functional deterioration, in which a diagnosis "dementia" could not be made according to modified DSM-III-R/IV criteria. This usually involved persons with insufficient capacities to express themselves, e.g., by severe generalized motor impairment or severe chronic depression, or persons with a beginning dementia who did not meet DSM criteria during the study, but did afterwards.

Diagnostic Criteria

The following diagnostic criterion for a diagnosis "dementia," based on score-change as compared with original DMR scores, led to the best sensitivities and specificities.[11]

Table 3.3 Modified Diagnostic Criteria for Dementia (Modified DSM-III-R)[7,8]

A. Demonstrable evidence of decline of original level of short- and long-term memory
   (observed in daily circumstances)
B. At least one of the following (observed in daily circumstances)
   1. Disturbance of original level of spatial or temporal orientation
   2. Aphasia
   3. Apraxia
   4. Personality change
C. The disturbance in A and B significantly interferes with work for usual social activities or
   relationships with others
D. Not occurring exclusively during the course of delirium

An increase of the Sum of Cognitive Scores (SCS) of 7 points or more and/or an increase of the Sum of Social Scores (SOS) of 5 points or more, independent on the original level of ID. Results of application of this criterion are presented in Table 3.4.

A sensitivity of 100% means that all cases with an expert diagnosis of dementia will be correctly identified by the DMR. A specificity of 75% indicates that 75% of persons without dementia are correctly classified as "no dementia" by the DMR. However, 25% is incorrectly classified as "dementia" (the so-called false-positives). In such cases, further diagnostic assessment usually identified a functional deterioration by other conditions. Although of course a specificity of 100% would be preferable, this is in practice realized in hardly any diagnostic instrument.[12,13] Which specificity is acceptable, will vary per condition. For example, a false-positive diagnosis of cancer would have to be avoided as much as possible. However, in the case of dementia in persons with ID, a specificity of 75% is acceptable. Indeed, in a majority of cases with incorrect diagnoses of dementia, further diagnostic assessment resulted in relevant and often treatable other diagnoses (severe sensory impairments, severe motor impairments, severe physical disease, and psychiatric conditions). As a conclusion, with the DMR, functional deterioration as a result of cognitive as well as noncognitive aspects is identified. Longitudinal judgment of scorechanges is more reliable than single completion and is therefore preferable.

Results of the last evaluation suggested that the DMR is less accurate in case of specific causes of dementia, other than dementia in Alzheimer disease (DAD) (e.g., vascular dementia). However in this stage, such a conclusion can only be speculation because of the small subgroups.

Table 3.4 Sensitivity and Specificity of the DMR (95% Confidence Intervals Between Parentheses)[11]

	Sensitivity	Specificity
70+	7/7 (100%) (59–100)	19/26 (73%) (52–88)
DS	8/8 (100%) (63–100)	27/36 (75%) (58–88)

Judgment by Committee on Test Affairs Netherlands

The quality of the Dutch DMR has been recently rated by the Committee on Test Affairs Netherlands (COTAN) of the Dutch Institute of Psychologists. The purpose of these ratings is twofold. Test users are informed about the quality of available instruments, which information can help them in choosing an instrument. Besides, the ratings supply feedback to test-developers about the quality of their products. An English translation of the rating procedure has been published in the *International Journal of Testing*, 2001, pp. 155–182. Outcomes for the DMR (2B.13 DVZ) were as follows: theoretical basis and soundness of test development procedure, satisfactory; quality of testing materials, good; comprehensiveness of the manual, good; norms, satisfactory; reliability, satisfactory; construct validity, satisfactory; criterion validity, satisfactory.

Applications of the DMR

Dementia

The DMR has been designed in principle for the diagnosis of dementia in adults with ID. However in practice, because DAD is the most prevalent cause of dementia, we have primarily evaluated the sensitivity for DAD. Due to small subgroups, the sensitivity for rarer types of dementia has been evaluated insufficiently.

Early Detection

Our longitudinal evaluation shows, that in all cases, a diagnosis based on DMR scores was made prior to or at the same time as an expert diagnosis according to international criteria could be made (DSM-III-R/DSM-IV).

Screening Instrument and Effect Instrument

We stress that the DMR is not an instrument for a definite diagnosis of dementia, because severe progressive physical and other psychiatric conditions, or a combination of less severe conditions, may influence the scores as well. Therefore, the DMR has to be used as a screening instrument, i.e., for selection of persons for further specialist diagnostic assessment. Recently, the instrument has been proven satisfactory to evaluate effects of interventions.[14,15]

Repeated or Single Completion

The basis for a diagnosis of dementia is always a deterioration from the former individual level of cognitive functioning. Indeed, the DMR is most sensitive in case of multiple measures.

Originally, we have also tried to develop criteria for a single completion of the DMR, which would simplify large-scale screenings, e.g., in connection with research projects. This is only possible under the condition that reliable and interindividually comparable data from former intelligence tests, performed prior to any deterioration, is available. In our own evaluation studies, the participants' level of ID had been ascertained with several tests: Stutsman Mental Measurement of Preschool Children,[16] Peabody Picture Vocabulary Test,[17] and Leiter International Performance Scale.[18] The results may not be completely comparable to other scales, used nowadays and in other countries to test functional levels. Therefore, a diagnosis based on a single application of the DMR is now considered insufficiently valid, and is strongly discouraged by us.

Criteria for Persons to be Tested

The DMR is applicable to persons with mild, moderate, or severe ID (developmental ages around 2–10 years). It is not applicable to persons with profound ID (developmental age lower than 2 years) and to persons with severe ID (developmental age 2–3 years) combined with severe other disabilities, such as motor impairment or hearing loss. In such cases, DMR scores may approach extreme levels before any functional deterioration ("ceiling effect").

Who Answers the Questions?

The questionnaire has to be completed by a family or staff member who is familiar with the person. Carefulness and objectivity are very important. This may be advanced by DMR completion not by a single person, but by a family member together with a staff member, or by several carers together, and preferably guided by the investigator.

Who Interprets the Answers?

Interpretation of the results is only useful in combination with other diagnostic data, as applies for each diagnostic instrument. Therefore, this should be done by the diagnosing physician, psychologist, or behavioral therapist.

Directions for Diagnostic Use

Because longitudinal judgment of DMR scores provides the most reliable diagnosis, it is advised to routinely perform a first scoring of the DMR before any functional deterioration is observed. This might be done when somebody moves to a home for several persons with ID, or joins a day activity center. Any observed deterioration should prompt repeated completion of the DMR. If no scorechange is found, consistent with a diagnosis of dementia, further diagnostic assessments are to be aimed primarily at other causes of deterioration, such as a depression or sensory impairment. Dependent on the development of symptoms, a next DMR scoring and judgment is advised after 6–12 months.

In case of a DMR diagnosis "dementia," referral for specialized psychiatric and general physical examination is advised, according to national or international guidelines.[19–22] In any case, visual and hearing functions are to be actively tested, because of increased risks of age-related sensory impairments in this population, which are missed in many persons with ID.[23,24]

Rating

The questionnaire is provided with a simple linear score system, in which the items have three response categories: 0 points, no deficit; 1 point, moderate deficit; 2 points, severe deficit. The subject's behavior during the past 2 months has to be judged. If an item cannot be defined, e.g., in case of a lack of expressive capacities of the subject, the score has to be "2."

The items are clustered in eight subscales (Table 3.1) and placed in an arbitrary sequence, to prevent response tendencies. Combined scores on the first three subscales (short-term memory, long-term memory, and orientation) are indicated as the SCS. Combined scores on subscales four through eight (speech, practical skills, mood, activity and interest, and behavioral disturbance) as the SOS.

The questionnaire is provided with a short instruction for completion. Completion takes 15–20 min.

Other Studies of the DMR

Since the availability of an English translation of the DMR, it is clinically used in many countries around the world. Several researchers have evaluated the DMR for their country, or used it in epidemiological or intervention studies.

The DMR in Diagnostic Test Batteries

Since the 1990s, other diagnostic instruments, both informant-based and to be administered directly to persons with ID, have been applied or developed to assess for dementia. Most of these tests are aimed at specific symptoms, such as maladaptive behavior, memory decline, or verbal fluency, or are specifically designed for persons with DS. Combinations of such tests in diagnostic batteries have been recommended by several groups.[25–28] The DMR in all cases was presented as the most promising informant-based screening tool in most adults with ID, including those with DS. It is the only informant-based scale available for assessing orientation.[27]

Evaluations of the DMR

Evaluations by other authors concern mostly single completions of the DMR, referencing to Intelligence Quotient (IQ) levels. It appeared that such results were less satisfactory than in our own evaluations, probably due to application of varying tests for IQ or functional levels, or other criteria for levels of ID. For this reason, Prasher proposed for persons with DS in the United Kingdom modified higher cut-off scores for single DMR scores.[29]

Burt and colleagues(30) in the United States, specifically evaluating assessment of orientation in 138 adults aged 29–82 years, found fair to good agreement between DMR scores on the subscale "Orientation" (single ratings) and direct assessment. The level of agreement was negatively influenced by lower functioning, DS, and higher age.

Deb and Braganza[31] in the United Kingdom compared ratings on several informant-based scales with the clinician's diagnosis among 62 adults with DS. The diagnosis according to DMR criteria (single ratings) showed sensitivity and specificity at the .92 level for both categories. In this study, the observer-rated scales appeared more useful for the diagnosis of dementia than the used direct neuropsychological test.

Silverman and colleagues[32] performed a study of dementia in 273 adults with ID, applying multiple tests 18 months apart. As opposed to our own findings, single ratings of the DMR, referencing to IQ measurements with Wechsler Adult Intelligence Scale and Stanford–Binet scales earlier in adulthood, distinguished more effectively between individuals with and without dementia than score-changes during the study period. Sensitivity of scorechanges over the 14–18 month period was less impressive than reported in the DMR manual. However, we suspect that in this study, the dementia process in a number of cases might have started before the first rating. As a result, no predementia baseline data were available, as is recommended in the manual. The authors recognize this: "It might be worthwhile examining change in DMR scores for incident cases for whom a predementia baseline is available, and to rely more on single assessment scoring otherwise." In this study, effects of different IQ tests were also studied. Indeed, it appeared that the IQ testing procedure had a significant effect on classifications of nondemented participants ($p < .05$) and a nonsignificant effect in other dementia status groups, but the power was low.

Finally, Shultz and colleagues[33] in the United States and Canada evaluated several screening tools for dementia in a case-control study, with 38 matched participants with mild to profound ID in each group. Again, single ratings were used for the DMR, referencing to IQ measurements that were at least 5 years old, obtained with a variety of methods. Paired *t*-tests for both SCS and SOS ratings were highly significant, without correlating to gender, age, IQ level, or DS. In a logistic regression analysis of all tests used, the DMR SOS was the variable that best predicted group membership.

The DMR in Intervention Studies

Prasher and colleagues[14,15] used DMR scores as the primary outcome measures in a 24-week randomized controlled trial (RCT) of the cholinesterase inhibitor donepezil. The study group consisted of 27 persons with DS and mild or moderate DAD. There was a tendency that donepezil halted the rate of decline, but the sample size was too small for statistical significance. The trial was continued as an open-label study until a total of 104 weeks. Long-term use of donepezil significantly reduced the rate of decline ($p < .001$). A comparable 24-week effect study of rivastigmine has also been published by Prasher and colleagues.[34] Prasher concludes that the DMR is sufficiently sensitive to measure scorechanges as a result of intervention (personal communication 2004).

An uncontrolled evaluation of treatment with different cholinesterase inhibitors in a network of specialist memory clinics for people with ID in Southwest England was recently reported.[35] Here too, the DMR was used to monitor intervention effects, showing a significant deterioration of total scores in the last two assessments before treatment ($p < .01$), during a mean interval of 10.8 months. Treatment seemed to stabilize scores during a mean period of 7.4 months, whereas the SOS showed a significant improvement ($p < .05$).

Summary

Recently, the DMR has been rated satisfactory to good by the COTAN. From secondary studies by other authors, we conclude that the DMR is high-ranking in recommendations for diagnostic batteries.[25,26,28] Apart from cognitive items, it also scores noncognitive items. It is the only informant-based scale for assessment of orientation.[27] Authors use preferably single DMR ratings, requiring reliable IQ levels for referencing.[29,31–33] In that case, the choice of IQ tests or tests for functional levels may negatively influence sensitivity and specificity, because different tests lead to different dementia classifications based on the DMR.[32] Nevertheless, results in these studies are promising. Corroborated by the findings of Silverman and colleagues,[32] we stress again that a sensitive DMR diagnosis based on scorechanges requires baseline ratings prior to onset of dementia and not during dementia. The DMR is a sensitive instrument to monitor changes as a result of intervention.[14,15,35]

Our own evaluation studies have shown that the DMR is not sensitive in persons with profound ID, because of a "ceiling effect." To our clinical experience, there is a "bottom effect," too: in persons with very mild or borderline ID and beginning dementia, it may take years before DMR scores reach the level of a dementia diagnosis. Apparently, the DMR is not sensitive to more subtle functional deterioration, and the questions have been designed with capacities of people with moderate and severe ID (developmental ages 2–6 years) in mind.

During our evaluation studies, the DSM-III-R was replaced by the DSM-IV.[9] Did this influence the validity of the DMR? In the DSM-IV, some of the former clinical criteria for a diagnosis of dementia were omitted, namely "disturbances of abstract thought in judgment" and "personality change." According to the DSM-IV, deterioration from the original level of functioning has to be more explicitly taken into account. The only change in our modified criteria would therefore be the absence of the criterion "personality change" (Table 3.3). Because this aspect in practice has hardly played a decisive role in our specialist diagnoses, it is not to be expected that outcomes of our validity studies would have shown relevant changes by applying DSM-IV instead of DSM-III-R criteria.

In 1995, we participated in an international consensus group for diagnosis of dementia in people with ID, which advocated application of ICD-10 rather than DSM-IV criteria in this population.[25,26,36] The reason was that, as compared to the DSM-IV, in the ICD-10 more emphasis is placed on noncognitive aspects of dementia (e.g., emotional lability, irritability, and apathy). In practice, these noncognitive aspects are often the first signs, reported in individuals with ID, rather than cognitive aspects. The consensus group concluded that in this way a "two-step" diagnostic procedure is introduced, in which a possible diagnosis of dementia will be reconsidered, if observed behavioral changes are not accompanied by evidence of cognitive decline. It was seen as an advantage that in this way, consideration of all possible causes of decline is required, including of those that are treatable. These recommendations are in line with the more recent recognition of the role of psychiatric and behavioral disorders in dementia syndromes in clinical research in the general population.[37] Aylward and colleagues[26] observed that ICD-10 and DSM-IV overlap completely on the part of cognitive decline. The DMR was cited as a reliable method to detect a decline in memory and other cognitive abilities, a decline in emotional control or motivation, or a change in social behavior. Indeed, with the second part of the DMR, a range of noncognitive aspects can be assessed, among which the aspects, mentioned in the ICD-10.

We conclude that the distinction of "dubious dementia" and "dementia" in the expert diagnosis in our DMR studies is in fact comparable to this "two-step" procedure. Our choice to classify "dubious dementia" as "dementia" for the assessment of sensitivity and specificity is in line with the considerations of the international consensus group. Therefore, it may be assumed that evaluation of the DMR against a clinical diagnosis according to ICD-10 criteria would have resulted in comparable outcomes.

References

1. Evenhuis HM, Kengen MMF, and Eurlings HAL. (1998). Dementie Vragenlijst voor Verstandelijk Gehandicapten (DVZ). Tweede, geheel gewijzigde druk. Amsterdam: Harcourt Test Publishers.
2. Evenhuis HM, Kengen MMF, and Eurlings HAL. (2006). Dementia Questionnaire for People with Intellectual Disabilities (DMR). Amsterdam: Harcourt Test Publishers (orders through info@harcourt.nl or www.harcourt-uk.com).
3. Evenhuis HM. (1990). The natural history of dementia in Down's syndrome. Arch Neurol 47: 263–267.
4. Evenhuis HM. (1997). The natural history of dementia in ageing people with intellectual disability. J Intellect Disabil Res 41: 92–96.
5. American Psychiatric Association. (1982). Diagnostic and Statistical Manual of Mental Disorders, 3rd edn., revised. Washington DC: American Psychiatric Association.
6. McKhann G, Drachman D, Folstein M et al. (1984). Clinical diagnosis of Alzheimer's disease: Report of the NINCDS-ADRA Work Group. Neurology 34: 939–944.
7. Evenhuis HM, Eurlings HAL, and Kengen MMF. (1984). Diagnostiek van dementie bij bejaarde zwakzinnigen (diagnosis of dementia in ageing persons with ID). Ruit, multidisciplinair tijdschrift voor ontwikkelingsstoornissen, zwakzinnigheid en zwakzinnigenzorg 40: 14–24.
8. Kengen MMF, Eurling HAL, Evenhuis HM et al. (1987) Een onderzoeksinstrument voor de diagnostiek van seniele dementie bij zwakzinnigen (the Dementia questionnaire for mentally retarded persons: an assessment instrument for diagnosis of senile dementia in persons with mental retardation). Ruit 43: 24–30.
9. American Psychiatric Association. (1987). Diagnostic and Statistical Manual of Mental Disorders, 4th edn. Washington, DC: American Psychiatric Association.
10. Evenhuis HM. (1992). Evaluation of a screening instrument for dementia in ageing mentally retarded persons. J Intellect Disabil Res 36: 337–447.
11. Evenhuis HM. (1996). Further evaluation of the Dementia Questionnaire for Persons with Mental Retardation (DMR). J Intellect Disabil Res 40: 369–373.
12. Griner MF, Mayewski RJ, Mushlin AI et al. (1981). Selection and interpretation of diagnostic tests and procedures. Ann Int Med 94: 553–600.
13. Sacket DL, Haynes BR, Guyatt GH et al. (1991). Clinical Epidemiology: A Basic Science for Clinical Medicine, 2nd edn. Boston, MA: Little, Brown & Co.
14. Prasher VP, Huxley A, Haque MS et al. (2002). A 24-week, double-blind, placebo-controlled trial of donezepil in patients with Down syndrome and Alzheimer's disease—Pilot study. Int J Geriatr Psychiatry 17: 270–278.
15. Prasher VP, Adams C, Holder R et al. (2003). Long term safety and efficacy of donezepil in the treatment of dementia in Alzheimer's disease in adults with Down syndrome: Open label study. Int J Geriatr Psychiatry 18: 549–551.
16. Stutsman R. (1931). Mental Measurement of Preschool Children. Chicago: World Book Company.
17. Dunn LM. (1959). Peabody Picture Vocabulary Test. Washington, DC: American Guidance Service, Inc.
18. Leiter RG. (1969). Leiter International Performance Scale. Chicago: Stoelting Company.
19. National Institutes of Health. (1987). Differential diagnosis of dementing diseases. NIH Consensus Statement 6: 1–27.
20. Royal College of Psychiatrists. (1995). Consensus statement on the assessment and investigation of an elderly person with suspected cognitive impairment by a specialist old age psychiatry service. Royal College of Psychiatrists, Council Report CR 49, London, UK.
21. Centraal Begeleidingsorgaan voor de Intercollegiale toetsing (1997). Herziening consensus Diagnostiek bij het dementiesyndroom (Revised consensus Diagnosis of the dementia syndrome). CBO, Utrecht, the Netherlands.

22. Knopman DS, DeKosky ST, Cummings JL et al. (2001). Practice parameter: Diagnosis of dementia (an evidence-based review). Report of the Quality Standards Subcommittee of the American Academy of Neurology. Neurology 56: 1143–1153.
23. Splunder J van, Stilma JS, Bernsen RMD, and Evenhuis HM. (2005). Prevalence of visual impairment in adults with ID in the Netherlands: A cross-sectional study. Eye Sep 9; (Epub ahead of print).
24. Meuwese-Jongejeugd A, Vink M, Zanten B et al. (2006). Prevalence of hearing impairment in 1598 adults with an intellectual disability: Cross-sectional population-based study. Int J Audiol 45: 660–669.
25. Aylward EH, Burt DB, Thorpe LU et al. (1995). Diagnosis of dementia in individuals with intellectual disability. Report of the AAMR-IASSID Working Group for the establishment of criteria for the diagnosis of dementia in individuals with intellectual disability. Washington: American Association on Mental Retardation.
26. Aylward EH, Burt DB, Thorpe LU et al. (1997). Diagnosis of dementia in individuals with intellectual disability. J Intellect Disabil Res 41: 152–164.
27. Burt D and Aylward E. (2000). Test battery for the diagnosis of dementia in individuals with intellectual disability. J Intellect Disabil Res 44: 175–180.
28. Strydom A and Hassiotis A. (2003). Diagnostic instruments for dementia in older people with intellectual disability in clinical practice. Aging Mental Health 7: 431–437.
29. Prasher VP. (1997). Dementia questionnaire for persons with mental retardation (DMR): Modified criteria for adults with Down's syndrome. J Appl Res Intellect Disabil 10: 54–60.
30. Burt DB, Primeaux-Hart S, Phillips NB et al. (1999). Assessment of orientation: relationship between informant report and direct measures. Ment Retard 37: 364–370.
31. Deb S and Braganza J. (1999). Comparison of rating scales for the diagnosis of dementia in adults with Down's syndrome. J Intellect Disabil Res 43: 400–407.
32. Silverman W, Schupf N, Zigman W et al. (2004). Dementia in adults with mental retardation: Assessment at a single point in time. Am J Ment Retard 109: 111–125.
33. Shultz J, Aman M, Kelbley T et al. (2004). Evaluation of screening tools for dementia in older adults with mental retardation. Am J Ment Retard 109: 98–110.
34. Prasher VP, Fung N, Adams C. (2005). Rivastigime in the treatment of dementia in Alzheimer's disease in adults with Down syndrome. Int J Geriatr Psychiatry 20: 496–497.
35. Brown S, Mathurin W, McBrien J et al. (2004). A naturalistic study of cholinesterase inhibitors in adults with Down syndrome and dementia of Alzheimer type. In: 12th World Congress International Association for the Scientific Study of Intellectual Disability (IASSID), Montpellier.
36. World Health Organization. (1992). ICD-10: International Statistical Classification of Diseases and Related Health Problems, 10th revision. Geneva: WHO.
37. Ritchie K and Lovestone S. (2002). The dementias. Lancet 360: 1759–1766.

Chapter 4
Dementia Scale for Down Syndrome

E. Jozsvai, P. Kartakis, and A. Gedye

Introduction

The term "dementia" refers to deterioration in intellectual functioning or the development of multiple cognitive deficits affecting memory, language, comprehension, and activities of daily living. There are many types of dementia that occur in the general population and in those with intellectual disability (ID). Dementia in Alzheimer Disease (DAD) is the most common form of dementia in Down syndrome (DS). Its clinical manifestation increases with aging from 8%, in those between 35 and 40 years old, to approximately 22%, for those aged 40+. For individuals in the 60+ age group, the rate is estimated to be 69%.[1–3] Among institutionalized individuals with DS the rate of dementia has been reported to be as high as 88%.[4] However, other types of progressive dementia (e.g., vascular dementia), reversible dementias (e.g., untreated hypothyroidism), and conditions that mimic dementia also occur in adults with ID.[5] The pattern and symptoms of DAD in adults with DS are similar to those observed in the general population,[6] except that the decline in DS adults starts from a significantly lower level of functioning.

Unfortunately, most instruments for assessing dementia in the general population are unsuitable for use with the ID population, especially in persons with severe or profound ID. In recent decades there has been an increasing need for instruments (a) to assess for dementia in ID adults and (b) to aid differential diagnosis when cognitive decline presents.

Background on the Development of the Scale

The development of one such instrument, the Dementia Scale for Down Syndrome (DSDS)[7] began in 1987. First, the author identified some of the psychometric concerns critical in assessing this population, especially those in the severe or profound range of ID. These concerns included:

V.P. Prasher (ed.), *Neuropsychological Assessments of Dementia in Down Syndrome and Intellectual Disabilities*,
DOI: 10.1007/978-1-84800-249-4_4, © Springer Science+Business Media, LLC 2009

1. The need for information that does not rely on a person's performance on tests in a person unable to follow test instructions.
2. The need to distinguish features *typical* of that person from features that indicate *loss* of functioning.
3. The need to rate severity of dementia relative to the person's premorbid intelligence.
4. The need to consider conditions that cause a *reversible* dementia or *mimic* a dementia.
5. The need for *charting over time* to detect worsening of functioning or recovery of functioning (in the case of reversible dementia).

Gedye then designed a protocol that addressed those specific psychometric concerns. She collected longitudinal data over 8 years on adults with ID (with and without DS), then did a detailed item analysis, identified item patterns reflecting differential diagnoses, and developed a scoring system that reflects stages of severity of dementia. Thereafter, reliability and validity studies were conducted in a different province on 50 adults with DS.

In 1995, the DSDS was published. Since that time, many researchers have used this scale (including those in non-English countries such as Japan, Holland, and France) and some have published results on the psychometric properties of the scale (see "Psychometric properties of the DSDS"). The DSDS was standardized and validated mostly on adults in the severe and profound range of ID, but researchers have also used it with adults in the mild and moderate range of ID. Clinicians have more testing options when assessing adults in the mild or moderate range of ID because they can be given tests that require direct performance whereas those in the severe or profound range may never have been able to do such tests. Over the years, several observer-rated instruments have been developed for people with ID.[8–10] One of the earliest and perhaps most commonly used among these is the DSDS.

The Dementia Scale for Down Syndrome

The DSDS is a 60-item informant-based instrument that was designed to aid in diagnosing dementia in individuals with ID, especially those with DS. The DSDS can also be used to establish a baseline measure on individuals with ID who are at risk of developing dementia because of their age, but currently do not exhibit signs of cognitive decline. The scale is classified as a Level C test, thus clinical psychologists with experience in the psychometric assessment of ID are qualified to administer it and interpret the results. A psychometrist with an undergraduate degree and a minimum of 2 years experience with tests of intellectual and adaptive functioning may also qualify to administer the scale. The DSDS requires that caregivers responding to the questions know the person for at least 2 years and be familiar with the person's skills of daily living. It is recommended that two people be interviewed and, if the client works, to have one informant from the person's workplace. The DSDS is available commercially in English and French versions.

To detect the onset of dementia relative to baseline functioning, the DSDS includes many items that reflect losses in people with ID. Items on the DSDS can be rated as "typical" (if a feature is characteristic of the individual through his/her lifetime) or "not applicable" (if the feature was never part of the person's baseline cognitive or behavioral repertoire). It is important in assessing people with ID to ensure items of lifelong impairment are not misread as signs of dementia, and the DSDS was designed specifically to avoid psychometric confounding of lifelong impairments with dementia-related impairments in the list of items.

Items reflecting symptoms of dementia such as changes in interest and initiative, losses in verbal, spatial or temporal memory, decline in comprehension or language ability, may be rated "absent" or "present." The onset and progression of dementia is ascertained by tracking changes in functioning over time through follow-up assessments every 6–12 months. Questions are grouped into three categories with items that address "early stage," "middle stage," and "late stage" characteristics of dementia.

To meet criteria for the early stage, the person must have a minimum of three losses in the cognitive area and this is referred to as the Cognitive Cut-off Score (CCS). This helps eliminate people with many social/affective changes and/or physical losses—those who are perhaps depressed or showing physical declines—but who are not showing cognitive losses. It is also important to identify a time period when cognitive and other changes began. To do this, the DSDS user identifies the date of an early loss (often item #1) then typically adds 6 months to define a time period when early losses surfaced, thereby identifying the onset of dementia changes. (Occasionally the onset of dementia is very slow and the DSDS has provisions for initial changes to be spread over 12–18 months after the "first" sign of decline.) The criteria for early-stage dementia require at least three cognitive losses—a CCS of 3 or greater—and a total of ten changes taken from 20 possible early-stage items and 20 possible middle-stage items.

Screening for Conditions that Cause Reversible Dementia or Mimic Dementia

The DSDS aids in differential diagnosis by (a) listing clusters of test items that point to conditions that can co-occur, cause reversible dementias, or mimic dementia, and (b) providing additional questions to ask. The DSDS includes an easy-to-use section entitled Differential Diagnosis Screening Questions (DDSQ). This section covers possible signs of hypothyroidism, pain, vision changes, hearing changes, depression, medication-induced cognitive decline, sleep apnea, and vascular dementia. Most of these conditions are fairly common in older adults with DS. The DDSQ questions can assist the DSDS user to make further inquiries and/or provide information to physicians so that other possible diagnoses can be ruled in or out. Thus, the DSDS is useful for detecting reversible types of dementia, conditions that can mimic dementia, along with DAD and other progressive dementias. One DSDS test booklet provides space for recording changes in functioning over ten assessments.

Reversible Cognitive Deterioration

1. *Hypothyroidism* is one of the most frequent causes of reversible dementia. Approximately 60% of those with DS over the age of 35 years have abnormal thyroid functions.[11] Specific symptoms of hypothyroidism include reduction in energy, motivation, and a general decline in cognitive functioning, including memory and attention.
2. *Vitamin B$_{12}$ deficiency* can also cause forgetfulness, irritability, poor appetite, withdrawal, and a general functional decline. Symptoms of this form of dementia disappear once vitamin B$_{12}$ therapy is administered.
3. *Depression* can cause a reversible cognitive decline, but can also coexist with dementia, thus making differential diagnosis quite challenging in the DS population. It is one of the most commonly diagnosed psychiatric disorders in DS adults,[12–14] and it is frequently found to be related to the elevated rate of hypothyroidism common in the syndrome. Depression may be related to changes in the social milieu, such as death of parents or loss of residential caregivers. Presenting symptoms are likely to involve skill and memory declines, tearfulness, irritability, and a noticeable decrease in energy and activity level, loss of daily living skills, hallucinatory-like self-talk, and even psychotic features.[15–17] Urinary incontinence may be associated with depression in adults with DS, and this condition also occur in individuals with DAD.[18]
4. *Medication-induced cognitive decline* is another concern.[5,19] Gedye[7,19] described several cases of reversible dementia, and among those were cases related to seizure disorder or long-term use of neuroleptic medication. The history of cognitive decline in these cases ranged from 0.5 to 5 years, and they progressed to middle-stage features but did not progress to late-stage dementia. The majority of the individuals were under 40 years of age, but reversible dementia was also documented in adults over the age 50 years with DS and ID of other etiologies. After better seizure control or discontinuation of neuroleptic medication, all these individuals recovered their abilities.

Conditions that Can Mimic Cognitive Decline

1. *Sleep apnea* occurs in approximately 50% of DS individuals.[20] It may produce behavioral changes such as irritability, depression, or paranoia. In addition, ongoing sleep disturbance can result in a significant decrease in attention and concentration, and it can produce a decline in an individual's general cognitive ability.[21]
2. *Hearing and visual impairment:* Adults with DS are at greater risk for both auditory and visual impairment. It has been reported that 40% to 70% of adults with DS likely experience sensorineural and/or conductive hearing loss, and 46% develop cataracts.[22] These sensory impairments often produce behavioral changes such as withdrawal from regularly enjoyed activities and general apathy,[23] thereby mimicking a cognitive decline.

Psychometric Properties of the DSDS

In the standardization sample 60 individuals with DS (63% male and 37% female) aged 40 years or older were selected to participate in a longitudinal study of age-related cognitive changes. The participants were selected from a provincial (British Columbia, Canada) DS population of 229 people (56% male and 44% female) who were 40 years of age or older when the study began in 1987. Ten individuals with symptoms of dementia who were under the age of 40 years were also included in the DS group and were followed for several years. A control group of 47 non-DS elderly with ID was also followed. Levels of intellectual functioning, according to the DSM-IV criteria,[24] in the DS group included mild (1%), moderate (23%), severe (46%), and profound (30%) ranges. The percent distribution of levels of ID in the control group was comparable, with the least number of participants in the mild (5%) and profound (16%) categories, and the majority falling within the moderate (27%) and severe (51%) ranges. The demographics for the DS and the control group are presented in Tables 4.1 and 4.2.[7]

Reliability and Validity Studies

In the context of psychological testing clinicians are concerned with interrater reliability, the degree of agreement between results obtained by two independent raters administering the same test. An index of interrater reliability is the kappa coefficient.

Table 4.1 Demographic Characteristics of the DS sample

Cohort by year of birth	Number	Male	Female	Community (C) or institution (I)	
1919–1927	10	6	4	4 C	6 I
1928–1937	29	19	10	18	11
1938–1947	21	13	8	18	3
Subtotal	60	38 (63%)	22 (37%)	40 (67%)	20 (33%)
After 1947	10	4	6	10	0
Total	70	42 (60%)	28 (40%)	50 (71%)	20 (29%)

Table 4.2 Demographic Characteristics of the ID Control Group

Cohort by year of birth	Number	Male	Female	Community (C) or institution (I)	
1909–1917	3	2	1	2 C	1 I
1918–1927	10	6	4	4	6
1928–1937	19	9	10	14	5
Subtotal	32	17 (53%)	15 (47%)	20 (63%)	12 (33%)
After 1947	5	4	1	4	1
Total	37	21 (57%)	16 (43%)	24 (65%)	13 (35%)

In the standardization study of the DSDS,[7] two clinicians independently interviewed the same caregivers. The assessments took place within a few days of one another. The obtained kappa coefficient was .91 for the dementia classifications, thereby indicating a high interrater reliability for the DSDS.

Validity refers to the "truthfulness" of the instrument, or the degree to which the test measures what it claims to measure. Construct and criterion-related validity are most often of interest to clinicians in applied settings. The goal of construct validation is to determine whether or not test scores provide a good measure of a specific construct. In the case of the DSDS the construct being measured is progressive loss of cognitive ability, or dementia. Gedye[7] evaluated the construct validity of the DSDS from evidence pertaining to the onset and progression of dementia. In the DSDS standardization sample, of the individuals with DS who progressed to late stages, 100% had previously met the scale's criteria for early stages and criteria for middle stages. Further evidence for construct-related validity of the DSDS can be found in the study by Temple and colleagues[25] that involved 35 adults with DS between the ages of 29 and 67 years. The participants were assessed by the DSDS and a battery of neuropsychological tests that have been shown to discriminate between individuals with DS with and without dementia.[26] The participants were followed for a minimum of 6 months, and some were followed for a total of 3 years. All of the participants had completed multiple assessments with the DSDS and/or the neuropsychological test battery. Approximately 20% of the participants were diagnosed with early-stage dementia, and 6% with middle- to late-stage dementia. All of the participants who were assessed as having early-, middle-, and late-stage dementia showed a substantial decline on the neuropsychological tests and/or on the DSDS at follow-up.

Criterion-related evidence for validity demonstrates whether test scores are systematically related to outcome criteria, i.e., the presence or absence of dementia. In the 1993 Ontario study of the scale's psychometric properties, a psychiatrist highly experienced with working with adults with DS, rated the presence or absence of dementia in 50 older adults with DS independently from a psychologist (the author) very experienced using the DSDS, and this yielded a kappa coefficient of .81.[7] Criterion-related validity can be estimated by comparing the test instrument with a clinician's diagnosis, as in the above example, or with another test. In addition to using a kappa coefficient, validity can also be expressed as sensitivity and specificity of a test. The validity indexes of sensitivity and specificity can be expressed as percent agreement, and/or a kappa coefficient. Sensitivity is defined as the proportion, or the percent, of true cases (individuals with a disorder) correctly categorized by the test as having the disorder. Specificity is the proportion of true noncases (healthy individuals) correctly diagnosed as being unaffected. The probability of agreement between a clinician's diagnosis and a diagnosis derived from an instrument can also be expressed in terms of the positive and negative predicting power of the test. The positive predictive power of a test is the probability that the person with a disorder is identified by the test as having that disorder. Negative predictive power is the probability that a person without the disorder will be categorized by the test as not having the disorder (see Shultz and colleagues[27] for details of calculating these indexes).

In the standardization study of the DSDS, Gedye[7] compared the dementia ratings of two clinicians for 46 DS individuals, and found a sensitivity of 100% and a specificity of 98%. Deb and Braganza[28] compared clinicians' diagnoses of dementia using ICD-10 criteria[29] with diagnoses arrived at using the DSDS and the Dementia Questionnaire for Mentally Retarded Persons (DMR; Chapter 3).[30] Sixty-two adults with DS, aged 35 to 75 years with mild (22.6%), moderate (66%), and severe (11.4%) ID participated in the study. Twenty-six of these individuals were diagnosed by a clinician as having dementia and 36 were rated as nondemented. On the DSDS, 22 of the clinician-diagnosed demented participants met the criteria for dementia, but four of the participants who met criteria on the DSDS were not diagnosed by clinicians as demented. Thus, the comparison between the DSDS criteria and the rate of diagnosis of dementia by a clinician yielded a specificity of .89 and a sensitivity of .85. In contrast, the comparison between clinician diagnosis and the DMR criteria for dementia was .92 for both measures of sensitivity and specificity. A significant positive correlation ($r = .868$, $p < 0.001$) was found between overall scores on the DSDS and the DMR, and between DSDS scores and the main subcategories measured by the DMR ($r = .82$, $p < 0.001$).

Further support for the high sensitivity and specificity of the DSDS was provided by a study of 40 DS adults, aged 26 to 66 years.[31] The majority of these individuals were described as functioning within the moderate (85%) and mild (12.5%) ranges of ID. Baseline and 2-year follow-up assessments with DSDS were compared with a clinician's diagnosis of dementia using ICD-10 criteria. At baseline, values of sensitivity and specificity were 58% and 96%, respectively. Sensitivity increased to 75% at 2-year follow-up, and specificity remained at 96%. Thus, relative to a single administration, the diagnostic accuracy of the DSDS increased with repeat assessment. The disparity observed between the clinician's diagnosis and the DSDS rating occurred mostly in the cases of high-functioning individuals (mild to moderate range of ID), who showed early symptoms of dementia. But as dementia progressed from middle to late stages, there was a high agreement between the clinician's diagnosis and the DSDS.

Huxley and colleagues[31] argued that the DSDS has a lower diagnostic sensitivity for high-functioning individuals because it was originally designed to assess adults whose abilities fall within the severe and profound ranges of ID. However, with high-functioning individuals, caregivers may not notice the early signs of dementia because the initial symptoms are often indistinct. Oliver and Holland[32] conducted a review of several case reports of DS adults with Alzheimer's neuropathology and found that over 50% of the individuals had vague symptoms including depression, lethargy, and apathy. Evenhuis[4] similarly described symptoms of apathy, withdrawal, loss of self-help skills, and daytime sleepiness in a sample of adults with DS with early-stage dementia. These behavioral changes may be overlooked by caregivers, especially if contact with the rated person is infrequent. Also, most individuals with mild to moderate ID have attained a certain level of education and skill development, and therefore in the early stages of dementia they likely have the ability to compensate for skill loss, compared to their lower functioning peers. Research suggests that level of cognitive functioning may influence the expression of DAD in persons with DS and, similar to individuals without ID, higher functioning individuals with DS may experience a deferral of DAD symptoms.[25]

More recently, Shultz and colleagues[27] compared the DSDS with a number of other neuropsychological assessments: the DMR, the Reiss Scale, the Shultz Mini Mental Status Exam, and the Paired-Associate Learning Task. The authors investigated the relative efficacy of each test to differentiate demented from nondemented individuals. The participants were 38 adults (45% female and 55% male), between 45 and 74 years of age, with Intelligence Quotient (IQ) scores ranging from 20 to 71. Sixty-eight percent of participants had a diagnosis of DS. The participants were assigned to one of two groups based on a clinician's diagnosis of dementia or absence of dementia using DSM-IV[24] or ICD-10[29] criteria. The groups were matched on the following variables in order of priority: diagnosis of DS, age (within a range of 5 years), and IQ level (assessed 5 years prior to the study) within a 15-point range. The results showed that the DSDS and DMR significantly differentiated between the two groups. For both of these tests, scores were not significantly related to age, gender, IQ or the presence or absence of DS. The DSDS showed a sensitivity of .65 and a specificity of 1.0, whereas for the DMR the corresponding values were .65 and .93, respectively. The positive predictive power for the DSDS was 1.0 and its negative predictive power was .76. For the DMR a lower positive (.92) and negative (.70) predictive power was reported. Based on these findings the investigators concluded that the DSDS and the DMR are both "useful in distinguishing between groups with and without dementia; and it is difficult to state simply which instrument was more effective." The slightly better ability of the DMR to discriminate between the two groups was attributed to the relatively high proportion of high-functioning individuals in the sample.

While sensitivity and specificity are widely used measures of test validity, some investigators are skeptical about these indices. Ball and colleagues[8] argued that comparing a clinician's diagnosis with a screening test is a potentially problematic procedure. First there is no "gold standard tool to diagnose dementia in DS. Second, clinicians make clinical decisions using broadly the same assessment methods as these screening instruments" (p. 614), and thus high levels of agreement are likely, whether or not the assessments are valid. It is worth pointing out that the DSDS is not classified as a "screening tool" but a diagnostic instrument that was developed only after 8 years of longitudinal data were available on dozens of cases followed long enough to confirm progressive dementia (DAD) or not. Moreover, psychometric studies done on an independent sample from a different province were also done prior to its publication. These aspects do not make the DSDS a "gold standard," but do support its classification as a diagnostic tool, not a "screening" tool.

The DSDS in Neuropsychological Assessment

Alyward and colleagues[33] proposed that assessment of dementia in adults with DS requires the use of both caregiver interviews and direct assessment with psychometric instruments. To promote "state-of-the-art diagnostic practices and information exchange between clinicians and researchers," Burt and Aylward[34] recommended a battery of neuropsychological and adaptive behavior scales to be administered along with DSDS and/or other interview-based instruments. In response, the diagnostic sensitivity of a neuropsychological test battery in detecting dementia in adults with DS was evaluated.[26] The test battery consisted of Information and Orientation Questions, Block Design Test,[35] Fuld Object Memory Evaluation,[36] Grocery List, Boston Naming Test,[37] Peabody Picture Vocabulary Test—Revised,[38] and Test of Apraxia. The tests were administered to 35 individuals with DS to compare the group performance of older people with dementia (age 40–59 years), older people without dementia (age 40–66 years), and younger people without dementia (age 28–39 years). Dementia status of the participants was determined based on the DSDS diagnostic criteria. Participants in all three groups were within the moderate range of verbal ability. The most sensitive measures of dementia-related decline in the test battery were the Information and Orientation Questions and the Fuld Object Memory Evaluation. However, these neuropsychological tests could not be used in adults with ID in the profound range or many in the severe range. What instrument could be used with persons in the lower cognitive ranges? The DSDS is one such instrument as it was standardized on DS adults 76% of whom were in the severe or profound range plus the reliability–validity study done on a different group of DS adults 90% of whom were in the severe or profound range of ID.

Stanton and Coetzee[39] reported that the DSDS is a useful scale to include in a battery of tests to assess dementia in people with ID. Acquilano and colleagues[40] also included the DSDS in a battery of assessment tools for older adults with ID, and they mentioned that the DSDS is "sensitive for behavioral changes in the profound range of ID due to the manner of scoring" (p. 199).

Krinsky-McHale and colleagues[41] investigated age-related changes in memory functions relative to changes in memory that occur with early-stage dementia in DS. Eighty-five individuals with mild to moderate ID were administered a modified version of the Selective Reminding Test (SRT).[42] The participants were first tested with the SRT when they entered the study (baseline) and subsequently annually. Among the participants with DS, 14 cases (10 females and 4 males) were diagnosed by a physician as having dementia. The DSDS was completed for 13 of these individuals. Memory decline for the dementia group exceeded the decline expected with normal aging and was steeper than the decline exhibited by members of the nondemented group. In the dementia group, for 85% of the cases memory decline occurred several years before the DSDS criteria for early-stage dementia were met, or when the physician made the diagnosis of dementia. Furthermore, in the majority of cases, memory decline preceded other symptoms of dementia by more than 1 year, and in some participants in more than 3 years. Thus, for early identification of dementia in persons with mild to moderate ID, test batteries should incorporate measures of memory in addition to caregiver instruments and other tests in order to evaluate multiple cognitive domains.

Published Studies that Used the DSDS

A summary of studies that used the DSDS is presented in Table 4.3.

Advantages and Disadvantages of the DSDS

Over the past 10 years, a considerable amount of research has been dedicated to evaluate the efficacy of the DSDS. The psychometric properties of the DSDS are now well established. The merit of the scale is in its ability to detect and diagnose dementia in adults with DS, and to distinguish functional decline from other

Table 4.3 Summary of Studies Employing the DSDS to Detect Dementia in Adults with ID

Aylward et al.[43]	DSDS used to confirm MRI diagnosis of DAD
Burt and Aylward[34]	DSDS was found to be useful with adults with ID of etiologies other than DS; lists strengths and weaknesses of scale
Burt et al.[44]	DSDS used to aid in identification of dementia in cross-sectional design of aging in DS adults
Deb and Braganza[28]	Good positive correlation found between DSDS and DMR scores, and between DSDS and psychiatrist ratings
Devenny et al.[45]	DSDS used to classify severity of dementia
Devenny et al.[46]	DSDS used to support diagnosis of DAD
Huxley et al.[31]	DSDS scores from baseline and 2-year follow-up were compared; accuracy of diagnosis improved with repeat assessment when dementia progresses
Huxley et al.[47]	DSDS used to assess dementia status in DS adults being evaluated for frequency and severity of challenging behaviors
Jozsvai et al.[26]	DSDS used in conjunction with neuropsychological test battery to detect presence of dementia in DS adults
Kojima et al.[48]	DSDS was translated for use in Japan; stages of dementia were evaluated and compared to prevalence rates from previous studies
Krinsky-McHale et al.[41]	DSDS used to identify early-stage dementia status
Lott and colleagues[49,50]	DSDS used to monitor changes following the administration of donepezil in DS-DAD adults
Nelson et al.[51]	DSDS used as a criterion measure of dementia; research assistants were trained to administer and score DSDS via videotaped instruction
Shoumitro et al.[52]	DSDS used to support ICD-10 diagnosis of dementia in a study assessing the role of apolipoprotein E gene in DS-DAD
Shultz et al.[27]	DSDS and DMR were highly correlated; DSDS was useful discriminating dementia groups
Strydom and Hassiotis[10]	Reviews the properties of the DSDS, including sensitivity and specificity in single assessments
Temple et al.[25]	DSDS scores were combined with scores from a neuropsychological test battery to assign diagnosis and to code for symptom severity

conditions that mimic the clinical symptoms of dementia. Another strength of the DSDS is that it allows for the staging of dementia. By tracking the progression of functional decline, caregivers can plan for changing support needs, and physicians have the objective means to evaluate the efficacy of pharmacological interventions designed to slow and abate the clinical signs of dementia. The most frequent criticism of the DSDS is related to its reduced sensitivity to detect the earliest signs of dementia in individuals with mild to moderate ranges of ID. But this is not surprising for at the onset of dementia high-functioning individuals with DS, similar to individuals without ID, are often able to compensate for some loss of skills. More importantly, the DSDS was designed principally for ID adults in the severe or profound range and was standardized mostly on adults in those ranges, not in the mild and moderate range. Thus, it is no surprise if a scale is less sensitive in an area that it never claimed to cover.

The strengths and weaknesses of the scale, as cited in the research literature, are summarized in Table 4.4.

Recent research suggests that repeated neuropsychological testing combined with caregiver interview scales is the most promising approach to assess dementia in high-functioning individuals with DS. Improving diagnostic accuracy may lead future research to develop age-appropriate test norms for the DS population which are then used to evaluate the efficacy of currently available psychometric instruments.

Table 4.4 Advantages and Disadvantages of the DSDS

Advantages
- Useful in detecting presence of dementia in DS adults
- Differentiates typical from atypical functioning and records duration of symptoms
- Does not depend on direct patient participation
- Includes analysis of item patterns and screening questions for differential diagnosis
- Evaluates early, middle, and late stages of dementia
- Good sensitivity and specificity
- High interrater reliability
- Can be used in low-functioning adults (severe or profound ID), those with little or no speech, and/or those in late-stage dementia when other instruments are unsuitable
- Allows for diagnosis on initial assessment because it focuses on losses at time of assessment, unlike other instruments currently available
- Requires administration and interpretation by a clinically trained professional which reduces the risk of false-positive and false-negative diagnostic errors

Disadvantages
- Reduced sensitivity for mild and moderate ranges
- Recommended that only psychologists or psychometrists administer the scale (see above)
- Two reliable informants are recommended (not always practical)
- Scoring system is not simple
- Relies on retrospective data, in that informants are required to compare current to previous levels of functioning

Summary

The DSDS is an informant-based instrument that was designed principally for assessing dementia adults in the severe or profound range of intelligence, but has also been found useful for assessing adults in the mild or moderate range of intelligence. It has good psychometric properties as confirmed independently by other researchers. The scoring method provides a rating of severity, identifies when an individual progressed from one stage to another, and facilitates tracking recovery from reversible dementia or during treatment studies. The scale incorporates features to facilitate differential diagnosis. It is used by psychologists around the world in at least 19 countries. The restriction on it for use only by psychologists (and psychometrists) is intended to reduce misdiagnosis of intellectual decline by people untrained in assessing intelligence. The DSDS can detect dementia in adults with and without DS and can distinguish functional decline from other conditions that mimic the clinical symptoms of dementia.

References

1. Janicki MP and Dalton AJ (2000) Prevalence of dementia and impact on intellectual disability services. Ment Retard 38: 276–288.
2. Lai F and Williams RS (1989) A prospective study of Alzheimer disease in Down syndrome. Arch Neurol 46: 849–853.
3. Wisniewski HM, Silverman W, and Wegiel J (1994) Ageing, Alzheimer disease and mental retardation. J Intellect Disabil Res 38: 233–239.
4. Evenhuis HM (1990) The natural history of dementia in Down's syndrome. Arch Neurol 47: 263–267.
5. Gedye A (1998) Behavioral Diagnostic Guide for Developmental Disabilities. Vancouver, BC: Gedye Research and Consulting.
6. Jozsvai E (2005) Behavioral and psychological symptoms of dementia in individuals with Down syndrome. J Dev Disabil 12: 31–40.
7. Gedye A (1995) Dementia Scale for Down Syndrome. Vancouver, BC: Gedye Research and Consulting;
8. Ball SL, Holland AJ, Huppert FA et al. (2004) The modified CAMDEX informant interview is a valid and reliable tool for use in the diagnosis of dementia in adults with Down's syndrome. J Intellect Disabil Res 48: 611–620.
9. Hoekman J and Maaskant M (2002) Comparison of instruments for the diagnosis of dementia in individuals with intellectual disability. J Intellect Dev Disabil 27: 296–309.
10. Strydom A and Hassiotis A. (2003) Diagnostic instruments for dementia in older people with intellectual disability in clinical practice. Aging Ment Health 7: 431–437.
11. Dinani S and Carpenter S (1991) Down's syndrome and thyroid disorder. J Ment Defic Res 34: 187–193.
12. Collacott RA, Cooper SA, and McGrother C (1992) Differential rates of psychiatric disorders in adults with Down's syndrome compared with other mentally handicapped adults. Br J Psychiatry 161: 671–674.
13. Myers BA and Pueschel SM (1991) Psychiatric disorders in persons with Down syndrome. J Nerv Ment Dis 179: 609–613.
14. Szymanski LS (1988) Integrative approach to diagnosis of mental disorders in retarded persons. In: Stark JA, Menolascino FJ, Albarelli MJ et al. editors. Mental Retardation and Mental

Health: Classification, Diagnosis, and Treatment Services. New York: Springer-Verlag, pp. 124–139.

15. Burt DB, Loveland KA, and Lewis KR (1992) Depression and the onset of dementia in adults with mental retardation. Am J Ment Retard 96: 502–511.

16. Lazarus A, Jaffe RL, and Dubin WR (1990) Electroconvulsive therapy and major depression in Down's syndrome. J Clin Psychiatry 51: 422–425.

17. Warren AC, Holroyd S, and Folstein MF (1989) Major depression in Down's syndrome. Br J Psychiatry 155: 202–205.

18. Pary R (2002) Down syndrome and dementia. Ment Health Aspects Dev Disabil 5: 57–63.

19. Gedye A (1998) Neuroleptic-induced dementia documented in four adults with mental retardation. Ment Retard 36: 182–186.

20. Stebbens VA, Dennis J, Samuels MP et al. (1991) Sleep related upper airway obstruction in a cohort with Down's syndrome. Arch Dis Child 66: 1333–1338.

21. Galley R (2005) Medical management of the adult patient with Down syndrome. J Am Acad Physician Assistants 18: 45–52.

22. Keiser H, Montague J, Wold D et al. (1981) Hearing loss of Down syndrome adults. Am J Ment Defic 85: 467–472.

23. Jozsvai E (1999) Alzheimer disease and Down syndrome. In: Brown I, Percy M, editors. Developmental Disabilities in Ontario. Toronto, ON: Front Porch Publishing, pp. 401–408.

24. American Psychiatric Association (1994) Diagnostic and Statistical Manual of Mental Disorders, 4th edn. Washington, DC: American Psychiatric Publishing.

25. Temple V, Jozsvai E, Konstantareas M et al. (2001) Alzheimer dementia in Down's syndrome: The relevance of cognitive ability. J Intellect Disabil Res 45: 47–55.

26. Jozsvai E, Kartakis P, and Collings A (2002) Neuropsychological test battery to detect dementia in Down syndrome. J Dev Disabil 9: 27–34.

27. Shultz J, Aman M, Kelbley T et al. (2004) Evaluation of screening tools for dementia in older adults with mental retardation. Am J Ment Retard 109: 98–110.

28. Deb S and Braganza J (1999) Comparison of rating scales for the diagnosis of dementia in adults with Down's syndrome. J Intellect Disabil Res 43: 400–407.

29. World Health Organization (1994) The ICD-10 Classification of Mental and Behavioural Disorders: Diagnostic Criteria for Research. Geneva: WHO.

30. Evenhuis HM (1992) Evaluation of a screening instrument for dementia in ageing mentally retarded persons. J Intellect Disabil Res 36: 337–347.

31. Huxley A, Prasher V, and Haque M (2000) The dementia scale for Down syndrome (letter to the editor). J Intellect Disabil Res 44: 697–698.

32. Oliver C and Holland AJ (1986) Down's syndrome and Alzheimer's disease: A review. Psychol Med 16: 307–322.

33. Aylward EH, Burt DB, Thorpe LU et al. (1997) Diagnosis of dementia in individuals with intellectual disability. J Intellect Disabil Res 41: 152–164.

34. Burt D and Aylward E (2000) Test battery for the diagnosis of dementia in individuals with intellectual disability. J Intellect Disabil Res 44: 175–180.

35. Wechsler D (1974) Wechsler Intelligence Scale for Children—Revised. New York: Psychological Corporation.

36. Fuld PA (1977) Fuld Object-Memory Evaluation. New York: Albert Einstein College of Medicine.

37. Kaplan EF, Goodglass H, and Weintraub S (1983) The Boston Naming Test. Philadelphia, PA: Lea & Febiger.

38. Dunn LM and Dunn LM (1981) Peabody Picture Vocabulary Test—Revised. Minneapolis, MN: American Guidance Service.

39. Stanton L and Coetzee R (2004) Down's syndrome and dementia. Adv Psychol Treat 19: 50–58.

40. Acquilano JP, Davidson PW, and Janicki MP (2006) Psychological services for older adults with intellectual disabilities. In: Jacobsen JW, Malick JA, Rojohn J, editors. Handbook of Intellectual and Developmental Disabilities. New York: Springer, pp. 189–207.

41. Krinsky-McHale SJ, Devenny DA, and Silverman WP (2002) Changes in explicit memory associated with early dementia in adults with Down's syndrome. J Intellect Disabil Res 46: 198–208.
42. Buschke H (1973) The Selective Reminding Test. J Verb Learn Verb Behav 12: 534–550.
43. Aylward EH, Li Q, Honeycutt NA et al. (1999) MRI volumes of the hippocampus and amygdala in adults with Down's syndrome with and without dementia. Am J Psychiatry 156: 564–568.
44. Burt DB, Primeaux-Hart S, Loveland KA et al. (2005) Aging in adults with intellectual disabilities. Am Ment Retard 110: 268–284.
45. Devenny DA, Krinsky-McHale SJ, Sersen G et al. (2000) Sequence of cognitive decline in dementia in adults with Down's syndrome. J Intellect Disabil Res 44: 654–665.
46. Devenny DA, Zimmerli EJ, Kittler P et al. (2002) Cued recall in early-stage dementia in adults with Down's syndrome. J Intellect Disabil Res 46: 472–483.
47. Huxley A, Van-Schaik P, Witts P (2005) A comparison of challenging behavior in an adult group with Down's syndrome and dementia compared with an adult Down's syndrome group without dementia. Br J Learn Disabil 33: 188–193.
48. Kojima M, Ikeda Y, Kanno A et al. (2000) Prevalence of dementia in institutionalized individuals with Down syndrome in Japan. J Intellect Disabil Res 44: 351.
49. Lott IT and Head E (2001) Down syndrome and Alzheimer's disease: A link between development and aging. Ment Retard Develop Disabil Res Rev 7: 172–178.
50. Lott IT, Osann K, Doran E et al. (2002) Down syndrome and Alzheimer disease: Response to donepezil. Arch Neurol 59: 1133–1136.
51. Nelson L, Orme D, Osann K et al. (2001) Neurological changes and emotional functioning in adults with Down syndrome. J Intellect Disabil Res 45: 450–456.
52. Shoumitro D, Braganza J, Norton N et al. (2000) APOE e4 influences the manifestation of Alzheimer's disease in adults with Down's syndrome. Br J Psychiatry 176: 468–472.

Chapter 5
The Dyspraxia Scale for Adults with Down Syndrome

A.J. Dalton

Introduction

Dyspraxia consists of a partial loss of the ability to perform purposeful or skilled motor acts in the absence of paralysis, sensory loss, abnormal posture or tone, abnormal involuntary movements, incoordination, poor comprehension, or inattention.[1] The existence of dyspraxia is usually tested by having the patient perform some motor act on command or by imitation.

Dyspraxia is a characteristic feature of dementia in Alzheimer's disease (DAD) in the general population, but it has been reported less frequently in persons with Down syndrome (DS). More typical changes in language and communication,[2] reduced speech output and gait deterioration,[3] bradykinesia,[4] and difficulty with walking unaided[5] have been reported in patients with DS with a clinical diagnosis of DAD. Impairment in walking abilities were reported in only 7 of 35 (17%) adults with DS, aged 35–65 years, for whom there was postmortem confirmation of a neuropathological diagnosis of Alzheimer disease (AD).[6]

The infrequent reports of dyspraxia attributable to DAD in persons with DS may reflect the difficult problems associated with the assessment of DAD in this population,[7–10] the lack of appropriate tests, and/or the difficulties in making effective observation and analysis of human movement.[11]

Rationale

The purpose of the Dyspraxia Scale for Adults with Down Syndrome is to provide a research tool for the evaluation of simple sequences of voluntary movements expected to deteriorate with the onset and progression of DAD among persons at all levels of premorbid intellectual disability (ID). The psychometric properties of the scale suggest it may also be useful for longitudinal research studies. The scale also holds promise as a primary outcome measure for measuring changes in cognitive functions in clinical trials involving aging persons with DS. It taps the abilities to perform simple sequences of highly practiced voluntary movements which are involved in the skills

V.P. Prasher (ed.), *Neuropsychological Assessments of Dementia in Down Syndrome and Intellectual Disabilities*,
DOI: 10.1007/978-1-84800-249-4_5, © Springer Science+Business Media, LLC 2009

of daily living. However, it does not attempt to measure those verbal and communication skills which would normally require a level of intellectual function outside the range of perhaps as much as one-third of all individuals with DS.

Background

The Dyspraxia Scale for Adults with Down Syndrome was an outgrowth of experience with the Western Aphasia Battery (WAB) developed by Kertesz and his associates at the University of Western Ontario in London, Ontario.[12] The WAB was designed to evaluate praxis in patients suffering from strokes[13] and later for hospitalized patients with clinical diagnoses of DAD.[14] Details are provided elsewhere of the adaptation of the WAB into a 48-item assessment tool called the Video-recorded Home Behavioral Assessment (VHB).[15,16] The VHB was used as the primary outcome measure in a clinical trial conducted to evaluate the effectiveness of intramuscular injections of desferrioxamine in slowing the decline in cognitive functions in patients with moderate severity DAD over a 2-year treatment period.[15] The VHB was used as the starting point for the development of the Dyspraxia Scale for Adults with Down Syndrome.

Dyspraxia Scale Construction

Several criteria were employed in the design of the Dyspraxia Scale for Adults with Down Syndrome. Each item selected for the Dyspraxia Scale had to meet the following criteria:[1] It required only a few seconds (2–5″) to perform on verbal request. [2] It was easy to administer.[3] It was easy to score.[4] It was easy to record permanently on video-tape.[5] It consisted of a sample of behavior which would normally be expected to occur in the daily life of the individual.[6] It could be easily modeled or demonstrated by the Examiner.[7] It was age appropriate.[8] It possessed adequate psychometric properties. The Scale was not designed as a speed test. Thus, no timed items were included nor were there any penalties for slow responses. The overall strategy was to construct a scale that would reflect the best possible performance under optimal conditions from individuals being examined. Simple instructions were used. The evaluations were conducted in environments with minimal stress, such as the individual's group home, shared apartment, workshop, day treatment center, or an office which was most familiar to the individual being tested. Scoring had to be straightforward (pass or fail), response definitions had to be explicit and unambiguous. Scoring by students or direct care staff had to be easy and reliable. Training of Examiners had to be brief but effective enough to meet a high standard set by an experienced Examiner. Items were also limited to those which required minimal verbal skills, language comprehension, and which could be performed by following simple verbal commands or by imitation of the Examiner. The aim was to create a scale that would be useful throughout the course from early to advanced DAD for individuals with levels of premorbid ID ranging from mild to profound.

The structure and scoring methods for the Dyspraxia Scale for Adults with Down Syndrome are similar to those of the VHB. The Scale is divided into three parts. Scores range from 4 (maximum) to 0 (minimum) for each item. It is recommended that Z scores be calculated based on means and standard deviations for each part of the Scale and for a total score to permit comparisons with Z scores obtained on other tests by the individuals being examined. See the report by Dalton and his colleagues[17] which documents the value of using Z scores when other tests are used alongside with the Dyspraxia Scale for Adults with Down Syndrome.

Description and Administration of the Dyspraxia Scale for Adults with Down Syndrome

Test Materials

The test materials used for Part 1, items #1 to 10 require no special test materials. It is important for safety reasons to provide something that the individual can lean on for support during attempts to perform the leg lift items (#11 and 12) such as a desk, cabinet, or chair. Items #14 to 20 require a sheet of white paper (letter size), pencil, scissors (medium size), a paper clip (1.75″ or 4.6 cm slightly bent to facilitate handling), three dimes, a small jar with screw-cap lid and a large, yellow, baseball cap. The materials for Part 2 (items 27 to 40) consist of a red silk rose with a 12″ semirigid plastic stem and two plastic green leaves attached 4″ below the flower, a 4″ black plastic comb, a packaged toothbrush (adult size), a teaspoon (white plastic), a hammer (small, 10″ handle), a medium-sized padlock (about 1″ diameter) with key, a one-ounce jam jar with lid, pair of cotton garden gloves with elasticized wrist (large size), standard letter-size white typing paper. These test items should be kept in a convenient briefcase or similar container on a chair beside the Examiner. The coins used in the Coin Task of Part 3 (test items #59 to 62) consist of two pennies, two nickels, two quarters, and two dimes. When used in non-United States or Canada locations, coins of the appropriate size and familiarity to persons living in these countries should be substituted for US coins. During test administration the test case containing the test materials can be placed on a chair within easy reach of the Examiner.

Detailed Scoring of the Dyspraxia Scale for Adults with Down Syndrome

Two methods were adopted for scoring. The first gives credit of 4 points for any successful response to each item, with or without "prompting," and "0" for failure on the item with or without prompting. The second method includes partial scores using prompting. Prompting consists of a graded increase in the amount of "assistance" which is provided by the Examiner to facilitate performance of the correct response by the individual being tested following a failure to perform correctly using simple verbal instructions repeated only once or twice. Prompting reduces the risk of incorrectly giving someone a "0" score for reasons unrelated to impaired praxis. This is achieved by reducing the dependence on verbal comprehension of instructions and minimizing the impact of sensory impairments, particularly hearing losses. Partial scores for incomplete responses using prompting methods are credited as follows:

4 points: A 4-point score is given for a correct response on request without any additional verbal prompts, imitation or modeling, or any form of physical assistance by the Examiner. Four points are assigned if the person correctly completes the item following the first or second request within 5–8 s.

3 points: Providing additional verbal cues and verbal hints to the person is referred to as verbal prompting. Successful performance after the use of verbal prompts decreases the score from a maximum of 4 points (unassisted) to 3 points.

2 points: Failure to obtain a correct response with verbal prompts signals the Examiner to use the next level of prompting that is, modeling. Successful performance by the individual following a modeling prompt is assigned a score of 2 points. A modeling prompt is a display by the Examiner of how the correct response should be executed. Modeling is performed when the previous verbal and gestured prompts have failed to elicit the requested behavior. The modeling is accompanied by the following verbal remarks: "Mr./Mrs...., watch me.... (e.g., make a fist, salute, etc.). Now, you do it, just like I did."

1 point: If modeling fails, then the Examiner uses "physical prompting." Physical prompting is a form of "hands-on" assistance provided by the Examiner to determine whether or not the person can perform the requested item with the addition of proprioceptive and tactile cues associated with passive movement. It is used when previous prompts have failed. It represents an attempt to make the task as easy as possible by providing the maximum number of visual and auditory cues now combined with tactile/proprioceptive cues as well. Three types of physical assistance are defined and used: (1). hand-over-hand in which the Examiner may place his/her hand over the person's hand that is holding the lid of the jar and help the person to turn the lid passively above the hand holding the open jar. (2) Moving the person in the situation requiring standing, sitting, or walking. The Examiner may place his/her hand under the person's elbow to provide support in standing up or sitting down. (3) Doing something for the person. Following the physical prompt the Examiner removes the contact and observes whether or not the person continues with the task to successful completion. A score of 1 point is given if the person can perform on his/her own.

0 points: Two attempts are made using physical prompting before discontinuation of the item and assignment of a score of 0 points. The individual must seem to be totally unresponsive, uncooperative, unable or unwilling to perform the required response.

Scoring Sheet

The scoring sheet (see Appendix 3) is divided into columns displaying the three parts of the Dyspraxia Scale for Adults with Down Syndrome with abbreviated descriptions of each test item. There is provision for entering the name, sex, date of birth, date of the examination, location, age, and the name of the Examiner.

Detailed Administration

Part 1: Psychomotor Skills: This section consists of 20 test items. Items 1 to 13 are administered while the individual is standing. Items 14 to 20 are performed at a desk or table while the Examiner and the participant are seated. All 20 items of Part 1 are scored on the basis of decreasing independence, as defined above. It is important to use verbal approval at the end of each response such as, "That's good," or "that's fine," or "Good work," etc.

- Item 1. "Walking." The person is instructed to walk toward the Examiner (or toward a tripod-mounted video camera if one is being used). Score of 4 points for independent walking upon single command or with only 1 or 2 repetitions of the same instruction. Score of 3 points for performance with verbal prompt of encouragement. Score of 2 points for correct imitation of the model (Examiner) with: "This is what I want you to do." Score of 1 point is given if physical assistance is used such as supporting arm and elbow while providing verbal encouragement with, "If I help you a little, try to walk toward the desk (or camera)." A person who uses a cane or walker is automatically scored 1 point. Score of 0 points if the person is unable, unwilling or refuses to complete the item. An individual who routinely uses a wheel chair automatically scores 0 points on this item.
  Following item 1, the next 12 items are administered while the individual is standing. The scoring is the same as for item 1.
- Item 2. "Standing." The person must be able to stand unassisted for 2–5 s.
- Item 3. "Look up." The individual must use his/her eyes or head to look up. A verbal prompt such as, "Look up at the ceiling," reduces the score to 3 points.
- Item 4. "Bend your head." The individual must lower his/her head toward the floor upon command for a score of 4 points. Use of the verbal prompt such as, "bend your head down," or "look at the floor," reduces the score to 3 points.
- Item 5. "Bow from the waist." The individual must bend slightly (2–3 in.) or completely from the waist. The use of the verbal prompt such as, "take a bow," reduces the score to 3 points
- Item 6. "Clap your hands." The individual must bring his/her hands together to indicate in front of the Examiner.
- Item 7. "Lift one arm over your head." A 4-point response includes lifting the arm straight up in the air near the head, placing the hand on the head, raising the hand behind the head.

- Item 8. "Lift the other arm over your head." A 4-point response is for behavior similar to that shown during the preceding item with the other arm.
- Item 9. "Turn your head to one side." The individual needs to keep his/her body facing forward, toward the Examiner (camera), while he/she turns the head to the side. Idiosyncratic behavior such as rotating the torso is acceptable. If the person is unable to perform this item correctly with one or two repetitions of the command, a correct, 3-point, response can usually be emitted with the verbal prompt, "look at the wall."
- Item 10. "Turn your head to the other side." The individual needs to keep his/her body facing forward toward the Examiner (camera) and turn the head to the side opposite to the one in Item 9. Again idiosyncratic variation is acceptable.
- Item 11. "Lift one leg." The individual should raise the leg off the floor and hold it in the air for at least 2 s. A score of 1 point is given if the person needs to place his hand a chair, desk, or cabinet provided for this purpose.
- Item 12. "Lift the other leg." The individual must raise the other leg and hold in the air for about 2 s for a full score of 4 points. A score of 1 point is given if the person places his hand for support on a chair, desk or cabinet intended for this purpose.
- Item 13. "Sitting." Upon completion of item 12, the individual is requested to sit at the table or desk (pointing by Examiner in the appropriate direction may be helpful) where the remainder of the test items are presented. This item is scored on the basis of the level of independence required to comply.
- Item 14. "Draw a circle." The individual is provided with a standard letter-size sheet of white paper and a pencil. A circle anywhere from 4 to 15 cm in diameter is acceptable for 4-point score as long as the response is performed with verbal command only with 1 or 2 repetitions. Three points are scored if verbal suggestions are required. If the Examiner needs to model the correct response a fresh sheet should be placed in front of the individual. The Examiner slowly draws a circle of about 10 cm (about 4 in.) in diameter in the upper half of the page and hands over the pencil to the individual with the instruction, "Now you do it, just like that, just like I did." The sheet is removed and stored as data for future analysis while the Examiner provides brief verbal approval.
- Item 15. "Draw a straight line." A new sheet of paper is placed in front of the individual. Instructions and scoring for this item are similar to item 14. At the end of the item, both the pencil and the paper are retrieved and put aside while the Examiner provides verbal approval to the individual.
- Item 16. "Clip two sheets." Two new letter-sized sheets of paper are placed side-by-side in front of the individual who is handed a large paper clip already somewhat bent outwards along one length to facilitate response. The instructions are: "Now, clip these sheets together with the clip." The individual is allowed about 30–45 s to complete the task. If necessary then, verbal prompts are provided such as: "put the sheets together. Put the clip on one sheet first, then put the other sheet under it." If modeling is required, the 2 sheets and clip are retrieved from the individual and the Examiner slowly demonstrates how to perform the task. Hand-over-hand assistance on this task is sometimes difficult.

At the end of this item the materials are retrieved and set aside while the Examiner says, "That's good. That's fine."

- Item 17. "Cut this paper sheet." A new letter-sized sheet of white paper is placed on the table along with a medium-sized pair of scissors with the instructions, "Now, I want you to cut this sheet of paper with the scissors." A score of 4 points is given if the individual performs correctly within 30–60 s. The sheet can be cut lengthwise, sideways, in half, or in one- to two-thirds fractions as long as no further prompting other than 1 or 2 repetitions of the same instruction. At the time the materials are retrieved the Examiner says, "Good. That's fine."
- Item 18. "Three coins with one hand." A small (one ounce) transparent jam jar is placed in front of the individual with three coins beside the jar (three dimes) with the request. "Please place each of the coins inside the jar." If the individual shifts hands during the task, the person is instructed not to do so. Picking up the coins with the thumb and the fingers or sliding the coins to the edge of the table before picking them up are acceptable responses. At the end of this item the Examiner says, "That's fine. Good," and empties the coins back onto the table with the jar next to the coins and proceeds to item 19.
- Item 19. "Three coins other hand." A repeat of item 18 but now the person must successfully perform with the other hand. Trial is terminated with verbal approval by the Examiner while the items are removed and set aside at the same time.
- Item 20. "Put on the cap/take it off." An adult size baseball cap is placed on the table in front of the individual with the instruction: "Put the cap on your head." After completion, the Examiner says, "Yes. That's good. Now, please take it off." The cap is set aside while the Examiner again provides verbal approval.

Part 2: Apraxia: These items are also administered while the person is seated at a desk in an arm-chair or in a wheel chair. For bed-ridden patients who are awake and reasonably cooperative, every effort should be made to obtain responses to as many test items as possible to help in the identification of preserved skills. About 2–4 s are allowed for each response. Each response is immediately followed by brief verbal approval from the Examiner with remarks such as those used with the previous items. Rules for defining and scoring independent performance, verbal, physical prompting, and modeling are the same as described earlier. Verbal approval after each response is also provided for each item.

- Item 21. "Make a fist." The individual must independently clench his fingers and thumb into a fist. The hand should be off the table. The shape of the fist should be roughly "rounded" with allowance for various idiosyncratic positions of the thumb.
- Item 22. "Salute." The person is required to independently raise either hand to his forehead with or without the thumb tucked in the palm. Once the hand is clearly positioned the person then should swing the hand out and away from the head for a full score. Allowance should be made for individual differences in execution.
- Item 23. "Wave good-bye." The person must hold either the right or left hand in the air and wave the hand from side to side or in an up and down motion independently for a full score.

- Item 24. "Scratch your head." The person must independently raise the hand to the head and use fingers to scratch back and forwards at least once for full score. Allowances for individual differences in response topography should be made.
- Item 25. "Snap your fingers." The person must independently snap the middle finger against the thumb with or without a sound.
- Item 26. "Close your eyes." The person must independently shut either of his eyes so that no part of the eyeball is visible. The eye closure should be visible to the Examiner (and/or camera).
- Item 27. "Sniff a flower." The person must independently hold the flower (silk rose with petals and 8″ stem) within 1–2 in. of the nose and appear to sniff the flower by holding it there momentarily.
- Item 28. "Use a comb." The person must independently hold the comb and make the appropriate stroking movements over the head. It is not necessary that the comb go through the hair. A new comb should be used with each individual being tested.
- Item 29. "Use a toothbrush." The person must independently hold the toothbrush in either hand and make either up and down or side to side movements with the brush held with the bristles toward the face near the mouth. A new brush should be presented with each new participant.
- Item 30. "Use a spoon." The person must independently pick up the spoon (soup size) from the table with either hand and bring it up toward the mouth. The person may or may not make a scooping motion with the spoon for a full score.
- Item 31. "Use a hammer." The person must pick up the hammer placed on the table in front of him/her and make one or two downward motions with the head of the hammer pointed downwards.
- Item 32. "Use a key." A small key is placed in front of the person. The person must independently pick up the small key from the table and make turning motions in the air to pretend opening a door.
- Item 33. "Open a jar." After a small (one ounce) jar with a screw cap is placed in front of the person, a full score is obtained if the person independently unscrews the lid using both hands, following verbal request only.
- Item 34. "Close the jar." The person gets a full score for replacing and screwing the lid back on the small jar without prompting. If placed incorrectly or too loosely the Examiner then proceeds with the prompting procedures outlined above and scores accordingly.
- Item 35. "Put on the (right hand) glove." An adult-size right-hand glove is placed in front of the person with the verbal request, "please put this on." Full credit is given if the person responds correctly without prompting. All fingers should be in their proper place. This is checked by the Examiner by reaching over and feeling through the glove for the finger positions. The person is then asked to remove the glove.
- Item 36. "Put on the (left hand) glove." The person is required to independently put on the left hand glove after removing the glove from the right hand following performance of item 35.

- Item 37. "Unlock a padlock." A small padlock and key are placed side-by-side and the person gets a full score if he/she independently picks up both items, inserts the key in the key hole and turns the key until the lock opens. An allowance of about 30 s is given before giving additional prompting procedures.
- Item 38. "Lock the padlock." The Examiner presents the lock with the key still inserted in position and with the swivel open. The person is required to independently swivel the catch until it is over the hole of the padlock then to press down firmly until the catch snaps shut. About 30 s are allowed before introducing prompting procedures.
- Item 39. "Fold a sheet of paper." The person must fold the paper (8.5″ by 11″ ordinary typing paper) neatly in half, with the edges of both sides meeting within 2–3 cm of each other. There must be a visible crease in the fold of the paper produced by the appropriate hand movement. The direction of the fold makes no difference in the scoring.
- Item 40. "Fold the paper again." Using the same folded paper, the person gets a full score for independently making a second fold in the sheet following instruction to do so without additional prompting.

Part 3: Body Parts/Coin Task: This part of the scale consists of 18 items adapted from the WAB and 4-coin identification tasks. Items 41 to 58 involve pointing to various parts of the body in response to simple verbal instructions. Each response is scored as either correct (4 points) or incorrect-unable-unwilling (0 points). The instructions can be repeated up to two times for a complete score. No prompting methods are employed for these items. Therefore, there are no partial scores for items in Part 3. However, as for all of the previous items, each response is immediately followed by brief verbal approval from the Examiner such as, "Good," or "that's fine," etc. These contingent verbal responses by the Examiner provide immediate feedback to the individual and also provide a cue indicating termination of the trial for each item, a useful feature if video recordings are involved in the test session.

The Examiner instructs the seated individual as follows: "Mr./Ms…., I am going to ask you to point to different parts of your body." The person is then requested to: "Point to your ear (item 41), nose (item 42), eye (item 43), chest (item 44), neck (item 45), chin (item 46), thumb (item 47), ring finger (item 48), index finger (item 49), little finger (item 50), middle finger (item 51), right ear (item 52), right shoulder (item 53), left knee (item 54), left ankle (item 55), right wrist (item 56), left elbow (item 57), and right cheek (item 58).

Immediately after item #58 of Part 3, the Examiner places eight coins (two pennies, nickels, dimes, and two quarters) in a random order on a letter-sized sheet of white paper within easy reach of the person. The person is then asked to, "Please give me a…" penny (item 59), nickel (item 60), quarter (item 61), and a dime (item 62). Each response is scored as either correct (4 points) or incorrect-unable-unwilling (0 points). The instructions can be repeated once or twice for a full score. No prompting methods are employed for these items. After the individual places a coin in the Examiner's hand, the coin is replaced on the sheet of paper and the coins are briefly shuffled on the page. Each response is immediately followed by brief verbal approval from the Examiner such as "Good," or "That's fine," etc.

Psychometric Properties of the Dyspraxia Scale for Adults with Down Syndrome

Validity and Reliability

Do the behaviors which are sampled in the Dyspraxia Scale for Adults with Down Syndrome constitute a representative sample? Do they include enough items or are there others which would be more intimately associated with the onset of DAD among persons with DS? It is not possible to answer these questions directly without postmortem studies of brain specimens from individuals who have died after performing the test as it is presently constructed. Thus, interpretation of the test scores obtained using this test must be cautious. It is assumed that the relatively large number of items in the Scale provides some protection against the likelihood of obtaining invalid measures. False conclusions can be minimized by careful adherence to a follow-up strategy in which baseline scores are compared with subsequent performances. Confidence in the conclusions is substantially increased by evidence of deterioration in scores. Improvements in scores over a short period of time could reflect a "practice effect" which is a characteristic of other tests of cognitive functions as suggested by Sano and her colleagues.[18] By the same token deterioration in performance scores at follow-ups are more likely to reflect true deterioration rather than fatigue, inattention, or lapses in concentration by the person being examined because of the relatively large number of test items.

Validity

The VHB, the predecessor of the Dyspraxia Scale for Adults with Down Syndrome, revealed an average decline in overall scores of 39.4%, from an average of 91.7% correct at baseline to 52.3% correct at a 2-year follow-up among 48 patients from the general aging population with a clinical diagnosis of mild to moderate severity AD.[15] This not only represents a clinically significant change but also demonstrates validation of the VHB against clinical diagnoses. Demonstration of similar changes in a group of persons with DS aged 54.4 years (SD = 2.62, min/max = 50/58 years) with a mean premorbid IQ = 39 points (SD = 14.1, min/max = 29/49 points) at the start, from a mean of 77.0% (SD = 6.35) correct dyspraxia items to 62.0% (SD = 28.73) correct over a 3.4-year period provides indirect evidence of the validity of the Dyspraxia Scale for Adults with Down Syndrome in persons with DS[19] because 48 of the 62 items of the Dyspraxia Scale were the same as in the VHB. However, since clinical diagnoses were not available for the participants with DS in this study[19] the declines in dyspraxia scores could also be attributed to so-called "normal aging" rather than to early DAD. However, the "normal aging" explanation of the results with persons with DS appears unlikely because the changes observed in the aging DS group occurred over a relatively short time period (about 42 months) and a group of "elderly" persons with mental retardation without DS (mean age = 72 years, min/max = 71/84 years at the start) in a separate study[19] with the Dyspraxia Scale for Adults with Down Syndrome showed no changes in scores over the same 3.4-year test period. Moreover, Devenny and her colleagues[20] have described as "normal aging" a slow decline of less than 1% per year in the performances on a test of selective reminding and a speeded psychomotor task across test times of up to 6 years in persons with DS older than 50 years of age. Needless to say, ultimate validation of the Dyspraxia Scale for Adults with Down Syndrome as a test of DAD in persons with DS needs the support of good clinical diagnoses and neuropathological diagnoses at postmortem.

Test–Retest Reliability

In one study,[21] 15 individuals (10 men, 5 women) including 9 with ID without DS and 6 with DS, with an average age of 61.9 years (SD = 14.26, min/max = 35/80 years), participated in a test–retest evaluation of the 62-item Dyspraxia Scale for Adults with Down Syndrome. Each individual was tested by the same Examiner on two occasions separated by 8 weeks. The percent agreement between first test and second test on an item-by-item basis was calculated for each participant. This analysis showed an overall average percent agreement on 84.4% of the items (SD = 11.30, min/max = 69.4/100%). This level of agreement compared favorably with the results of a similar analysis of item-by-item agreement of 78% which was obtained using the 48-item version of the Dyspraxia Scale for Adults with Down Syndrome (the VHB) which was employed in a previously published report involving 48 patients from the general aging population with diagnoses of mild to moderate severity DAD.[15]

In the second study,[19] the 62-item Dyspraxia Scale for Adults with Down Syndrome was administered twice to 25 individuals within a period of 3–6 weeks by a single Examiner. Test data were collected from 10 men and 6 women with DS (mean age = 46.1 years, SD = 8.12, min/max = 35/58 years) and from 6 men and 3 women with ID without DS (mean age = 71.1 years, SD = 4.71, min/max = 64/80 years). The first test scores for each of the 62 test items were compared with the retest scores on the same items for each of the 25 persons in an overall analysis using Statistica version 5.0 Statsoft software. The results indicated that the test–retest correlation exceeded $r = .96$,[19] thus indicating a high degree of test–retest reliability for the Dyspraxia Scale for Adults with Down Syndrome.

Test–Retest Reliability Over 3 Years

It is possible that scores on the Dyspraxia Scale for Adults with Down Syndrome would show progressive improvements with repeated testing due to practice effects over time. Scores could also show slow deterioration indicative of "normal aging." These possibilities were examined in an unpublished study described in the *Dyspraxia Scale for Adults with Down Syndrome Manual*.[22] The study was conducted on the Dyspraxia Scale Percent Correct items scores obtained on an annual basis over a 3-year period from 14 adults with DS (8 women and 6 men) with an average age of 45.9 years (SD = 5.55, min/max = 40/58 years) at the start. All were healthy. None showed any signs suggestive of early DAD as determined by direct care staff familiar with each individual throughout the period of the study. The average percent correct scores from the start, year 1, year 2, and year 3, were, respectively, 82.4% (SD = 7.18, min/max = 72/93), 84.5% (SD = 9.38, min/max = 68/95), 82.8% (SD = 10.24, min/max = 64/97),and 85.5% (SD = 9.64, min/max = 70/99). The results suggested that there were no improvements in scores reflecting a "practice effect" of repeated testing over the 3-year interval. Moreover, the absence of significant deterioration in scores was consistent with the report by Devenny and her colleagues[20] where she describes as "normal aging" the small magnitude of annual (1%) changes in cognitive scores over a 6-year follow-up of adults with DS.

Split-Half Reliability

The first time scores on the 62 items of the Dyspraxia Scale for Adults with Down Syndrome were divided into two sets of 32 scores with even-numbered items in set 1 and odd-numbered items in set 2. This was done for each of 140 adults with DS which included 109 from the standardization sample plus 31 additional individuals with DS who were referred to a clinic. The data were collected over a 2-year period by several Examiners. A split-half reliability coefficient was calculated using Statistica Version 5.0 Statsoft software. No cases were deleted from the analysis because there were no missing data. The analysis yielded a reliability coefficient of $r = .98$ for even versus odd items. These results raise the possibility of constructing alternate forms of the Dyspraxia Scale for Adults with Down Syndrome by using half of the test items in each form.

Internal Consistency: Cronbach's Alpha

Data from two studies were analyzed.

(i) **Study 1:** The first time Dyspraxia Scale for Adults with Down Syndrome scores from a group of individuals with DS ($n = 140$) collected at various care provider agencies in rural and suburban New York State were subjected to an item-by-item analysis to determine the contribution of each item to the overall Dyspraxia score. The data from 109 cases in the standardization sample (40 women and 69 men) were combined with data from 31 adults with DS who were referred to a Staten Island clinic for evaluation of possible DAD. Most were diagnosed with DS on the basis of chromosomal studies of blood specimens while the remainder of the individuals were diagnosed on a clinical basis. None had significant mobility or sensory impairments. None had seizures or psychiatric symptoms which were not adequately controlled by medication. Nineteen (26.0%) of the individuals were classified with premorbid mild ID. Ten (13.7%) of the individuals were classified with premorbid profound ID while the remainder had scores either in the moderate or severe range of ID.

(ii) **Study 2:** Data on the Dyspraxia Scale for Adults with Down Syndrome from 315 persons with DS were assembled and analyzed from seven independent investigators residing in Texas, Staten Island, Boston, Birmingham England, Manhattan, and Saskatoon, Saskatchewan. The analyses included data from 162 women and 153 men ranging in age from 33 to 77 years. Premorbid ID levels were available from the records of 262 of the 316. The sample included those with borderline ($n = 2$), mild ($n = 37$), moderate ($n = 137$), severe ($n = 75$), and profound ($n = 11$) levels of ID, respectively. Clinical diagnoses of DAD were reported for 41 and clinical diagnoses of no-DAD were reported for 57. Diagnoses for the remainder were not available. Table 5.1 is a summary of the results of both studies.

Test item number is shown in the first column. The second column is a short description of each item. The third column shows the mean dyspraxia scores for each of the 62 items from Study 1. The fourth column shows the standard deviation (SD) for each item from Study 1. No similar data were available from Study 2 for this analysis. The item-to-test correlations for each item for Study 1 and for Study 2 are shown in columns 5 and 6. Cronbach's alpha values with each item deleted from the test are shown for Study 1 in column 7 and for Study 2 in column 8. Cronbach's alpha with item deleted is never less than .92 in Study 1 and is .98 in Study 2. The very high alpha values for all of the dyspraxia items in Study 2 reflect the impact of the large sample size used for the analysis. When the two studies are viewed side-by-side it is convincingly evident that the Dyspraxia Scale for Adults with Down Syndrome has a very high degree of internal consistency.

Factor Analysis

A factor analysis of Dyspraxia Scale for Adults with Down Syndrome data collected from Study 2 involving 315 adults with DS was performed in order to examine some of the structural features of the Scale. Eigenvalues were calculated and estimates of the variance associated with each component were determined. There were nine components that exceeded 1.000. These eigenvalues and the contribution

Table 5.1 Test of Item-by-Item Internal Reliability: Study 1 and Study 2

Item No.	Short description of item	Study[a] Mean	SD	Item-to-test correlation Study 1	Study 2	Alpha with item deleted Study 1	Study 2
Part 1: Psychomotor skills: while standing							
1	Walking	3.94	0.73	.50	.54	.94	.98
2	Standing	3.91	0.58	.51	.54	.95	.98
3	Look up	3.51	1.34	.73	.67	.95	.98
4	Bend your head	3.52	1.48	.77	.72	.94	.98
5	Bow from the waist	3.32	1.68	.77	.70	.94	.98
6	Clap your hands	3.81	1.30	.79	.76	.94	.98
7	Lift one arm	3.36	1.35	.77	.76	.94	.98
8	Lift other arm	3.51	1.32	.82	.76	.94	.98
9	Turn head to one side	3.32	1.37	.66	.75	.95	.98
10	Turn head to other side	3.49	1.40	.76	.78	.94	.98
11	Lift one leg	3.65	1.38	.80	.76	.94	.98
12	Lift other leg	3.79	1.31	.76	.73	.95	.98
13	Sitting	4.37	1.60	.52	.58	.95	.98
Part 1: Psychomotor skills: while seated							
14	Draw a circle	3.65	1.40	.76	.75	.94	.98
15	Draw a straight line	3.53	1.54	.52	.69	.95	.98
16	Clip two sheets	–	–	–	.61	–	.98
17	Cut paper sheet	3.90	1.49	.66	.72	.95	.98
18	Three coins (one hand)	3.89	1.09	.58	.66	.95	.98
19	Coins (other hand)	3.78	1.30	.65	.71	.95	.98
20	Put on cap/take it off	3.95	1.04	.71	.67	.95	.98
Part 2: Apraxia							
21	Make a fist	3.33	1.52	.74	.73	.95	.98
22	Salute	3.20	1.55	.74	.67	.95	.98
23	Wave good-bye	3.68	1.28	.82	.76	.95	.98
24	Scratch your head	3.61	1.74	.69	.76	.95	.98
25	Snap your fingers	2.77	2.17	.51	.62	.96	.98
26	Close your eyes	3.69	1.62	.42	.68	.96	.98
27	Sniff a flower	3.82	1.40	.80	.80	.95	.98
28	Use a comb	3.99	0.98	.68	.74	.95	.98
29	Use a toothbrush	3.85	1.15	.73	.74	.95	.98
30	Use a spoon	3.76	1.21	.66	.77	.95	.98
31	Use a hammer	3.74	1.25	.76	.82	.95	.98
32	Use a key	3.67	1.60	.80	.73	.95	.98
33	Open a jar	3.96	1.06	.65	.75	.95	.98
34	Close a jar	3.88	1.20	.75	.77	.95	.98
35	Put on right glove	3.81	1.42	.75	.73	.95	.98
36	Put on left glove	3.81	1.43	.73	.73	.95	.98
37	Unlock padlock	3.54	1.54	.78	.77	.95	.98
38	Lock padlock	3.39	1.61	.77	.76	.95	.98
39	Fold a sheet of paper	3.77	1.16	.78	.83	.95	.98
40	Fold sheet again	3.73	1.43	.79	.80	.95	.98

(continued)

Table 5.1 (continued)

Item No.	Short description of item	Study[a]		Item-to-test correlation		Alpha with item deleted	
		Mean	SD	Study 1	Study 2	Study 1	Study 2
Part 3: Body parts and orientation							
41	Point to your ear	3.56	1.76	.71	.72	.92	.98
42	Point to your nose	3.61	1.71	.61	.77	.93	.98
43	Point to your eye	3.64	1.79	.66	.78	.93	.98
44	Point to your chest	3.01	2.36	.59	.61	.93	.98
45	Point to your neck	3.33	2.11	.72	.72	.92	.98
46	Point to your chin	3.35	2.33	.67	.63	.92	.98
47	Point to your thumb	3.41	2.14	.70	.65	.92	.98
48	Point to your ring finger	1.71	2.89	.30	.46	.93	.98
49	Point to your index finger	1.54	2.85	.12	.35	.93	.98
50	Point to your little finger	2.95	2.59	.67	.61	.92	.98
51	Point to your middle finger	2.13	2.89	.53	.51	.93	.98
52	Point to your right ear	2.89	2.55	.57	.50	.93	.98
53	Point to your right shoulder	2.88	2.82	.63	.52	.92	.98
54	Point to your left knee	2.98	2.79	.61	.51	.93	.98
55	Point to your left ankle	2.83	2.90	.69	.46	.92	.98
56	Point to your right wrist	2.34	3.06	.63	.43	.92	.98
57	Point to your left elbow	3.06	2.74	.49	.54	.93	.98
58	Point to your right cheek	2.81	2.83	.52	.53	.93	.98
Part 3: Coin identification task							
59	Give me a penny	2.96	2.45	.68	.66	.92	.98
60	Give me a nickel	2.86	2.88	.62	.55	.93	.98
61	Give me a quarter	2.96	2.58	.60	.63	.93	.98
62	Give me a dime	3.14	2.65	.75	.60	.92	.98

[a]No comparable data were available for study 2 at the time of this analysis.

of each component to the total variance are presented in Table 5.2. It can be seen that factor 1 accounted for 48.083% of the variance with factors 2 and 3 contributing 4.491% and 3.152%, respectively. These results are consistent with the idea that the Dyspraxia Scale for Adults with Down Syndrome is a one-dimensional scale.

Standardization—Normative Sample

Few, if any psychological or cognitive tests are effective in measuring functional impairment and deterioration throughout the course of DAD. Every test is likely to have either significant "ceiling effects" where the items are too easy or "floor effects" where the items are too difficult. As the dementing process progresses we must turn to direct observations of simple behaviors which are most likely to be

Table 5.2 Total Variance Explained in Factor Analysis

	Initial Eigenvalues		
Component	Total	% of Variance	Cumulative %
1	29.811	48.083	48.083
2	2.784	4.491	52.574
3	1.954	3.152	55.726
4	1.586	2.557	58.283
5	1.451	2.340	60.624
6	1.271	2.048	62.673
7	1.113	1.794	64.467
8	1.068	1.722	66.189
9	1.016	1.638	67.828

affected by AD.[21] Assessment of simple behaviors was the aim of the Dyspraxia Scale for Adults with Down Syndrome. However, no reference point was available for the test items selected. Therefore, in order to permit cross-test comparisons of changes over time with other cognitive tests it would be useful to know the distribution of dyspraxia scores of individuals with DS whose scores are representative of the general population of persons with DS without DAD. In addition, knowing the distribution and other characteristics of a "normative" sample of individuals with DS can provide a statistical basis for defining abnormality in terms of standard deviation units from the normative mean. A carefully selected sample of individuals was studied for this purpose.

First time Dyspraxia Scale for Adults with Down Syndrome scores from 122 adults with DS were reviewed for inclusion in a "standardization sample." Dyspraxia scores from 13 individuals were excluded for the following reasons. Four aging individuals (50, 53, 54, and 57 years of age at the start) were excluded (1 woman and 3 men) because they showed significant impairment of learning and memory functions as determined by performances on the Dalton/McMurray Visual Recognition Test,[23] a test used to detect the first memory changes associated with DAD in this population. The data from 9 of the 13 individuals (6 men and 3 women, 37–58 years of age) were excluded because 5 were uncooperative, one engaged in self-stimulatory behavior which interfered significantly with test performance, one was too young to be included (age of 12 years), and the Dyspraxia Scale for Adults with Down Syndrome was incomplete for 2 others. Each individual was involved on a regular basis in full- or part-time employment in a sheltered workshop, an industrial setting or day treatment program. There were 40 women and 69 men who met all of these criteria. The mean age of the women was 35.9 years (with SD = 10.48, min/max = 19/58 years) and for the men it was 34.9 years (with SD = 10.25 and min/max = 17/57 years). The mean intelligence quotient (IQ) scores for the women was 44 points (with SD = 15.1, min/max = 17/69 points) and for the men it was 37 points (with SD = 15.3, min/max = 16/66 points). There were no statistically significant differences between the women and men on any of the variables.

Consequently, the data for women and men were pooled to permit construction of norms. Conversion to Z scores for each person's performance is done using the familiar equation (percent correct score minus the standardization sample mean) divided by the standardization sample standard deviation for the parts and overall scores. Table 5.3 provides the basic data for conversion of raw dyspraxia scores into standard (Z) scores.

Standardization Sample—Part and Total Correlations

Table 5.4 provides a numerical summary of the Pearson Product Moment correlation coefficients for comparisons between the variables of age, Dyspraxia Scale for Adults with Down Syndrome Part 1, 2, 3, and overall scores. There were no statistically significant relationships between the dyspraxia scores and age. Parts 1 and 2 of the Dyspraxia Scale for Adults with Down Syndrome were more closely correlated with each other than with Part 3, reflecting difference in difficulty or the effect of a different factor. All three parts were highly correlated with the overall score.

Review of Published Research Studies with the Dyspraxia Scale for Adults with Down Syndrome

Dalton and Fedor[19] published the first study describing the development and standardization of the Dyspraxia Scale for Adults with Down Syndrome. The study also tested the hypothesis that older individuals with DS would obtain scores consistent with signs of the onset and progression of dyspraxia when compared with younger adults with DS. Persons with DS, 40 years of age and older showed statically significant deterioration which reflected "preclinical" signs of DAD. An older group with DS with "normal" dyspraxia scores at a mean age of 54.1 years, showed deterioration which began about 3.5 years later. The scores of a group between 40 and 49 years of age were indistinguishable from a younger group between 21 and 39 years of age. The results suggested that the onset of one of the early signs of DAD could be identified at an average age of 57.9 years among persons with DS using the Dyspraxia Scale for Adults with Down Syndrome.

Table 5.3 Descriptive Statistics for the Dyspraxia Standardization Sample ($N = 109$)

Statistic	Part 1	Part 2	Part 3	Overall
Mean	87%	88%	60%	78%
SD	13.60	15.27	24.27	15.83
Minimum	45%	20%	0%	23%
Maximum	100%	100%	98%	98%

84 A.J. Dalton

Table 5.4 Correlations Between Age and Dyspraxia Scores for the Standardization Sample

Variable	Age (years)	Part 1	Part 2	Part 3
Part 1	−.127	−		
Part 2	−.044	+.778	-	
Part 3	−.148	+.598	+.600	-
Overall	−.127	+.862	+.866	+.891

The aim of the same group of researchers in a further study[17] was to determine whether or not there was a specific sequence of cognitive changes over a 3-year period using three different tests. When compared with a young group of persons with DS (17–39 years at the start), an old group of persons with DS (40–58 years at the start) showed small but statistically significant changes over time suggestive of the "preclinical signs" of DAD. When the data were sorted into four subgroups on the basis of age, a more detailed analysis revealed that the subgroup that was 50 years of age and older at the start showed changes in scores which were of a magnitude more clearly indicative of early DAD. Deterioration in learning/memory scores on the Dalton/McMurray Visual Memory Test[23] began at a mean age of 54.2 years, followed later by deterioration in Dyspraxia Scale for Adults with Down Syndrome scores at a mean age of 56.9 years. Deterioration in ratings on a five-part, informant-based, maladaptive behavior rating scale, called the Multidimensional Observational Scale for Elderly Subjects (MOSES)[24] occurred at an intermediate age of 55.0 years. The results provided support for the hypothesis that persons with DS who are 50 years of age and older may develop a specific sequence of functional changes during the early stage of DAD. The possibility that those over 50 years of age showed deterioration because of between-group differences in the prevalence of one or more comorbid conditions which have a predilection for aging persons with DS was ruled out. None had a concurrent report of neurological, psychiatric, sensory or motor disabilities, other conditions and medications. These variables were routinely evaluated annually by knowledgeable nurses using a 35-item health checklist designed for the purpose.[17] The possibility that deterioration of the old DS subgroup could be due to a lower average level of ID was ruled out. Analysis of the IQ levels of the four subgroups revealed no statistically significant differences between them. The study also illustrated the value of using norms and standard scores (Z) to enhance the usefulness of a variety of tests to evaluate DAD in persons with ID.

A major challenge to developing therapeutic interventions for cognitive loss and DAD in aging individuals with DS is the selection of appropriate outcome measures. Sano and colleagues[18] describe the development and application of a short version of the Dyspraxia Scale for Adults with Down Syndrome called the Brief Praxis Test (BPT) as a primary outcome measure in a double-blind clinical trial with individuals with DS. Other tests to assess cognition, behavior, and clinical global function based on previous work in DS and in DAD were also used. Measures of cognition included verbal and nonverbal memory, vocabulary, and orientation. An informant-based measure of behavior and function was adapted from the MOSES[24] and the Dementia Questionnaire for Mentally Retarded

Persons (DMR)[25,26] for use with this group. This report also describes initial experiences using these measures with 108 participants (47 women and 61 men recruited into 20 research sites in five different countries) who were enrolled in the clinical trial. A diagnosis of DAD was made independently of the outcome measures. The level of ID was the best estimate of the highest lifetime functioning. The number of individuals at each level of ID was mild ($n = 23$), moderate ($n = 46$), severe ($n = 19$), profound ($n = 9$), and missing (n = 11). Mean BPT scores (out of a total possible 80 points) were 65.23 (SD = 12.14) and 58.72 (SD = 15.54), respectively, for those with a clinical diagnosis of no-DAD versus those with a diagnosis of DAD. Analyses of variance revealed highly significant association between BPT scores and level of ID (with $n = 98$, $F = 10.255$, $p < .000$) and BPT scores with diagnosis of DAD ($n = 107$, $F = 6.166$, $p < .015$).

As in other populations of persons with DAD, verbal learning, memory, and delayed recall scores proved to be highly associated with the presence of DAD in the study participants. With the exception of visual memory and orientation measures (which proved too difficult to use with portions of this cohort), the tests employed proved useful in the assessment of individuals across a range of premorbid levels of ID. The authors conclude that the measures chosen for the assessment of behavior and functional ability and the use of the Clinical Global Impression appear to be appropriate for this population and comparable to instruments that have captured pharmacological benefits in other disease groups.

Future Developments

The development of valid and reliable tests with high specificity and sensitivity for detecting DAD among persons with DS remains an important goal for the future. Almost of equal importance are tools that are highly sensitive to early changes in function. Short forms of the Dyspraxia Scale for Adults with Down Syndrome combined with a brief questionnaire should be explored in a variety of residential and clinical settings as a possible screening tool to raise the "level of suspicion" concerning the possibility of DAD. Detection of the early changes in cognition could "trigger" diagnostic referral and facilitate the planning of appropriate supports and care practices. Additional tests should be developed to tap other aspects of cognitive function. Some possibilities have been suggested elsewhere.[7,17] Evidence-based tests of cognitive function with adequate psychometric properties can make an important contribution to the diagnostic assessment process. Such tools can also provide a source of possible outcome measures for clinical trials aimed at evaluating the efficacy and safety of research medications that could alleviate and or prevent the onset and progression of DAD in this at-risk population. Outcome measures should be developed which can be used with persons at the severe and profound levels of ID because effectiveness of treatments may vary with this factor.

Validation of cognitive test performances requires correlation with postmortem examinations of brain tissue specimens. One important approach for conducting longitudinal clinical and neuropathological studies has been described by Visser and his colleagues.[27] Validation of the performances also requires correlation with clinical diagnoses using uniform criteria such as the ICD-10 of the World Health Organization or the DSM-IV of the American Psychiatric Association. The development work with the Dyspraxia Scale for Adults with Down Syndrome did not frequently include candidates recruited from diagnostic clinics. This practice means that a number of interpretations of declines in Dyspraxia Scale performances are plausible. Many morbid conditions have a higher than usual prevalence among older adults with DS. These include depression,[28] thyroid disorder,[29] the effects of stress and delirium,[29] psychiatric conditions,[30] and maladaptive behaviors.[31] However, where clinic facilities are available recruitment of research participants leads to a biased selection from a population likely to have some problems. Such a practice can introduce a serious limitation on the generalizability of the research findings. The development work with the Dyspraxia Scale for Adults with Down Syndrome rarely involved the selection of clinic samples. Persons with DS were recruited from a wide variety of settings (rural, urban, suburban, day treatment programs, workshops, small residential settings), different counties in New York State and in three different countries United States, Canada, and Britain). Thus, these samples are more likely to be representative of the population of persons with DS than clinic samples. However, without clinical evaluations, attribution of DAD as the cause of the observed declines in Dyspraxia performances must remain tentative.

The Dyspraxia Scale for Adults with Down Syndrome contains 62 items and administration can take up to an hour or so. Analyses reported above suggest that there is substantial "redundancy" in the test items. Such redundancy is important to minimize the effects of altered motivation, distraction, inattention, or momentary lapses in following instructions. A shorter version of the Dyspraxia Scale, called the BPT, consists of 20 items from the Dyspraxia Scale for Adults with Down Syndrome which can be administered in less than 10–15 min. The BPT was developed as a primary outcome measure for a randomized, double-blind, placebo-controlled trial of vitamin E.[17] Short versions of the Dyspraxia Scale, such as the BPT, could provide alternate forms useful for research applications involving repeated measures and it would shorten the length of time required for the examination of the individuals. Shorter test times would decrease the possible impact of fatigue and permit the addition of other tests as part of a less-fatiguing test session for the individual being examined.

Summary

The slow and insidious development of progressive dyspraxia is recognized as an early sign of DAD among aging persons from the general population. However, little is known about the age of onset, expression, and development of these AD-associated movement-related disorders among aging persons with DS. This report provides a brief description of the development of a 62-item Dyspraxia Scale for Adults with Down Syndrome. It includes the construction, administration, and scoring of the scale as well as the psychometric properties and the establishment of a standardization sample of 109 healthy individuals with DS. Analyses showed that the scale is highly reliable with high internal consistency of the items. A factor analysis involving a second sample of 315 individuals with DS from seven different sites is consistent with the idea that the Dyspraxia Scale for Adults with Down Syndrome is a one-dimensional scale. Other research reveals that deterioration over a 3-year period in scores among aging persons with DS 50 years of age and older is significantly greater than that shown adults with DS younger than 50 years of age. The results further indicate that the onset of clinically significant dyspraxia can be identified at an average age of 57.9 years among persons with DS. The significance and temporal relationships between changes in dyspraxia scores, in short-term recognition memory, and in maladaptive behavior ratings are also presented. Summaries of three published reports using the Dyspraxia Scale for Adults with Down Syndrome are provided and directions for the future are suggested.

Acknowledgments The development work on the Dyspraxia Scale for Adults with Down Syndrome, was supported by Surrey Place Centre, Toronto, Canada, the Ontario Ministry of Community and Social Services, a Medical Research Council of Canada grant MA-5364 to Arthur J. Dalton, Ph.D., an Ontario Health Research grant PR-633 to Donald R. Crapper-McLachlan, M.D., F.R.C.P.(C), University of Toronto, a USA NICHD grant RO1-HD08993 to Arthur J. Dalton, Ph.D., an NIA grant RO1-AG08849 to Arthur J. Dalton, a grant for Subproject 5 of NIA Program Project PO1-AG11531 with H.M. Wisniewski as Program Director, and NIA grant RO-1 AG-16381 to Arthur J. Dalton.

The generous contributions of the following investigators who provided Dyspraxia Scale for Adults with Down Syndrome data from their own work as part of Study 2 are also gratefully acknowledged: D.B. Burt, Ph.D., F. Lai, M.D., P.J. Patti, M.A., V.P. Prasher, M.D., N. Shupf, Ph.D., and L. Thorpe, M.D., Ph.D. Y.R. Chen, Ph.D., of the University of Texas, Houston, contributed the analysis of the internal consistency of Study 1. H.F. Andrews, Ph.D., of the New York Psychiatric Research Institute in Manhattan performed the statistical analyses of the internal consistency and a factor analysis of data from Study 2 of the Dyspraxia Scale for Adults with Down Syndrome.

The work would not have been possible without the cooperation and enthusiastic support of the staff, families, and friends of the following agencies in New York State: Pathfinder Village, Inc., Independent Group Home Living, Inc., Columbia County Arc, Young Adult Institute, O.D. Heck and Brooklyn Developmental Disabilities Services Offices, New York City Chapter of the New York State Association for the Help of Retarded Citizens. The support of the New York State Institute for Basic Research in Developmental Disabilities, Staten Island, New York, and the New York State Office on Mental Retardation and Developmental Disabilities are also gratefully acknowledged.

References

1. Lohr JB and Wisniewski AA (1987) Movement Disorders: A Neuropsychiatric Approach. Guilford Press, New York.
2. Orange JB and Zanon MV (2005) Language and communication in adults with Down syndrome and dementia of the Alzheimer type: A review. J Develop Disabil 12: 53–62.

3. Prasher VP (1995) Age-specific prevalence, thyroid dysfunction and depressive symptomatology in adults with Down syndrome and dementia. Int J Geriatr Psychiatry 10: 25–31.
4. Prasher VP (1995) Differential diagnosis between Alzheimer's disease and hypothyroidism in adults with Down syndrome. Downs Syndr Res Pract 3: 15–8.
5. Prasher VP and Filer A (1995) Behavioural disturbance in people with Down's syndrome and dementia. J Intellect Disabil Res 39: 432–6.
6. Dalton AJ and Crapper-McLachlan DR (1986) Clinical expression of Alzheimer's disease in Down's syndrome. Psychiatr Clin North Am 9: 659–70.
7. Aylward EH, Burt DB, Thorpe LU et-al. (1997) Diagnosis of dementia in individuals with intellectual disability. J Intellect Disabil Res 41: 152–64.
8. Oliver C (1999) Perspective on assessment and evaluation. In: Janicki MP and Dalton AJ (eds.). Dementia, Aging, and Intellectual Disabilities: A Handbook. Taylor & Francis, Philadelphia.
9. Burt DB and Aylward EH (1999) Assessment methods for diagnosis of dementia. In: Janicki MP and Dalton AJ (eds.). Dementia, Aging, and Intellectual Disabilities: A Handbook. Taylor & Francis, Philadelphia.
10. Prasher VP (2005) Alzheimer's Disease and Dementia in Down Syndrome and Intellectual Disabilities. Radcliffe Publishing, Oxford.
11. Ulrich DA, Riggen KJ, Ozmun JC et al. (1989) Assessing movement control in children with mental retardation: a generalizability analysis of observers. Am J Ment Retard 94: 161–8.
12. Kertesz A and Poole H (1974) The taxonomic approach to measurement of aphasic disability. Can J Neurol Sci 16: 1–7.
13. Kertesz A (1982) Western Aphasia Battery. Grune and Stratton, New York.
14. Kertez A (1994) Language deterioration in dementia. In: Emery VOB and Oxman TE (eds.). Dementia Presentation, Differential Diagnosis, and Nosology. Johns Hopkins University Press, Baltimore.
15. Crapper-McLachlan DR, Dalton AJ, Kruck TPA et al. (1991) Desferrioxamine in Alzheimer disease. Lancet 337: 1304–8.
16. McLachlan DR, Smith WL, and Kruck TP (1993) Desferrioxamine and Alzheimer's disease: Video home behavior assessment of clinical course and measures of brain aluminium. Drug Monitor 15: 602–7.
17. Dalton AJ, Mehta PD, Fedor BL et al. (1999) Cognitive changes in memory precede those in praxis in aging persons with Down syndrome. J Intellect Dev Disabil 24: 169–87.
18. Sano M, Aisen PS, Dalton AJ et al. (2005) Assessment of aging individuals with Down syndrome in clinical trials: Results of baseline measures. J Policy Pract Intellect Disabil 2: 126–38.
19. Dalton AJ and Fedor BL (1998) Onset dyspraxia in aging persons with Down syndrome: Longitudinal studies. J Intellect Develop Disabil 23: 13–24.
20. Devenny DA, Silverman WP, Hill AL et al. (1996) Normal aging in adults with Down's syndrome: A longitudinal study.. J Intellect Disabil Res 40: 208–21.
21. Dalton AJ (1992) Dementia in Down syndrome: Methods of evaluation. In: Nadel L and Rosenthal D (eds.). Down Syndrome and Alzheimer Disease. Wiley-Liss, New York.
22. Dalton AJ and Fedor BL (1997) Dyspraxia Scale for Adults with Down Syndrome. Manual, Available from first author. NYS Institute for Basic Research, 1050 Forest Hill Road, Staten Island, New York, 10314, email: daltonaj@aol.com
23. Dalton AJ and McMurray K (1995) The Dalton/McMurray Visual Memory Test. Bytecraft Inc., Waterloo, Ontario.
24. Dalton AJ, Fedor BL, Patti PJ et al. (2002) The Multidimensional Observation Scale for Elderly Subjects (MOSES): Studies in adults with intellectual disability. J Intellect Dev Disabil 27: 310–24.
25. Evenhuis HM, Kengen MMF, and Eurlings HAL (1990) Dementia Questionnaire for Mentally Retarded Persons. Hooge Burch Institute for Mentally Retarded People, Zwammerdam, the Netherlands.

26. Evenhuis HM (1992) Evaluation of a screening instrument for dementia in ageing mentally retarded persons. J Intellect Disabil Res 36: 337–47.
27. Visser FE, Aldenkamp AP, van Huffelen AC et al. (1997) Prospective study of the prevalence of Alzheimer-type dementia in institutionalized individuals with Down syndrome. Am J Ment Retard 101: 400–12.
28. Burt DB (1999) Dementia and depression. In: Janicki MP and Dalton AJ (eds.). Dementia, Aging, and Intellectual Disabilities: A Handbook. Taylor & Francis, Philadelphia.
29. Holland AJ (1999) Down's syndrome. In: Janicki MP and Dalton AJ (eds.). Dementia, Aging, and Intellectual Disabilities: A Handbook. Taylor & Francis, Philadelphia.
30. Thorpe LU (1999) Psychiatric disorder. In: Janicki MP and Dalton AJ (eds.). Dementia, Aging, and Intellectual Disabilities: A Handbook. Taylor & Francis, Philadelphia.
31. Prasher VP (1999) Adaptive behavior. In: Janicki MP and Dalton AJ (eds.). Dementia, Aging, and Intellectual Disabilities: A Handbook. Taylor & Francis, Philadelphia.

Chapter 6
Adaptive Behavior Change and Dementia in Down Syndrome: Case Classification Using the Adaptive Behavior Scale

W.B. Zigman, N. Schupf, T.K. Urv, and W. Silverman

Introduction

The history of Down syndrome (DS) and Alzheimer's disease (AD) is a long and complex one, with the first depictions of individuals with DS noted in artifacts almost 3500 years old.[1,2] In 1866, John Langdon Down[3] first used the scientifically incorrect and disparaging term "mongols" to describe a collection of symptoms he observed in almost 10% of the children he had treated at the Royal Earlswood Asylum, and in 1959, Lejeune et al.[4,5] discovered that DS was caused by triplication of the 21st chromosome. DS is the most frequent cause of genetically determined intellectual disability (ID) with a live birth rate of 1 in 733 births.[6]

Dementia is defined in the current edition of the *Diagnostic and Statistical Manual of Mental Disorders*[7] as the development of multiple cognitive deficits, involving memory, and aphasia (language impairment), apraxia (motor impairment), agnosia (perceptual impairment) or disturbance in executive functioning. Additionally, it is characterized by a substantial decline in adaptive abilities and significant functional impairment. Dementia in old age has been recognized since the time of Hippocrates,[8] however the specific neuropathology responsible for producing most cases was not identified until 1906, and the condition eponymously named AD.[9,10]

Clinical dementia in DS has been noted for over 100 years[11] and in 1948 Jervis[12] was the first to clearly describe the clinical and pathological characteristics of AD in three adults with DS. However, as recently as 30 years ago, the study of dementia in Alzheimer's disease (DAD) in individuals with DS did not attract much interest, given that relatively few individuals with DS lived long enough to develop signs and symptoms of dementia.[13] With the increasing graying of the world's population this is not the case, there could be 19 million adults over the age of 84 by the year 2050 in the United States alone,[13] and this has produced a proliferation of research on aging and the development of AD, and by extension, research on AD in DS.

V.P. Prasher (ed.), *Neuropsychological Assessments of Dementia in Down Syndrome and Intellectual Disabilities,*
DOI: 10.1007/978-1-84800-249-4_6, © Springer Science + Business Media, LLC 2009

91

Background to the Adaptive Behavior Scale

Adaptive behavior, defined as the "effectiveness of an individual in coping with the natural and social demands of his or her environment,"[14, p. 5] first became a formal component of the definition of ID in the late 1950s,[15-17] and today it remains an integral element of the diagnosis. Stated simply, the purpose of adaptive behavior assessment is to obtain an inventory of an individual's strengths and weaknesses.[18] The American Association on Mental Deficiency (recently renamed the American Association on Intellectual and Developmental Disabilities) Adaptive Behavior Scale (ABS) was first published in 1967,[19] and revised in 1974 (hereafter noted as ABS1),[20] and 1993 (hereafter noted as ABS2)[21] and was "designed to provide objective descriptions of an individual's adaptive behavior."[14, p. 5] While numerous additional adaptive behavior measures have been developed[22,23]; the ABS, in its various revisions has been well received and widely used within the field of ID.[18,24-26] Appendix 4 illustrates page 1 of the ABS1.

The classification of dementia in individuals with DS, compared with typically developing adults, is substantially more complex. Typically developing individuals can be expected to have baseline levels of functional abilities that are relatively invariant, while individuals with ID have preexisting impairments that may vary widely in their severity. To classify dementia for this latter population you must develop criteria that consider preexisting impairments, and document substantial declines from previous status. This chapter reviews the ways in which adaptive behavior, objectively measured using the ABS, has been applied to classify dementia in adults with DS. No published studies to date have used the ABS2 to classify dementia, possibly due to longitudinal nature of many of the studies reported, and the desire not to introduce experimental error by changing assessment instruments midstream. (The few studies that present similar findings for adults with ID without DS also will be presented.) First, descriptions of the ABS1 and ABS2 are presented, as well as their psychometric properties, followed by an overview of relevant studies that have used the ABS to examine dementia in DS. Finally, some relevant findings from our prospective study on aging and dementia in adults with ID with and without DS will be described along with suggestions for future research.

It should be mentioned that the classifications of dementia presented in the following studies do not constitute differential diagnoses of DAD. With current technology, the gold standard for diagnosis of DAD in adults with DS entails direct evidence of characteristic neuropathology rather than just the presence of dementia. However, given the virtually universal occurrence of AD-type neuropathology in adults with DS over the age of 40 years,[27] a clinical classification of dementia is tantamount to a differential diagnosis of DAD or together with another condition. These "mixed" cases are rare given that cerebral infarcts, one of the major alternative causes of dementia, are infrequent in adults with DS.[28]

Reliability and Validity of ABS

The ABS, in both its 1974 and 1993 versions, consists of two parts. Part 1 was designed to evaluate an individual's abilities and strengths in ten behavioral domains: (a) independent functioning, (b) physical development, (c) economic activity, (d) language development, (e) numbers and time, (f) domestic activity, (g) vocational activity, (h) self-direction, (i) responsibility, and (j) socialization. Interrater reliability coefficients for the ten domains in the ABS1 range from 0.71 (self-direction) to 0.93 (physical development), with a mean reliability coefficient of 0.86. Interrater reliability coefficients for the ten domains in ABS2 range from 0.88 (prevocational/vocational activity) to 0.99 (independent functioning and domestic activity), with a mean reliability coefficient of 0.95. Reliability of a Part 1 total score derived by summing the ten domain scores was estimated at 0.96.[29] (Table 6.1 displays the reliability coefficients for each adaptive domain for both the 1974 and the 1993 versions of the ABS.)

Part 2 of ABS1 was developed to evaluate an individual's maladaptive behaviors related to personality and behavior disorders, and contains 14 domains including: (a) violent and destructive behavior, (b) antisocial behavior, (c) rebellious behavior, (d) untrustworthy behavior, (e) withdrawal, (f) stereotyped behavior and odd mannerisms, (g) inappropriate interpersonal manners, (h) unacceptable vocal habits, (i) unacceptable or eccentric habits, (j) self-abusive behavior, (k) hyperactive tendencies, (l) sexually aberrant behavior, (m) psychological disturbances, and (n) use of medications (i.e., tranquilizers, sedatives, anticonvulsant drugs, and stimulants). Interrater reliability coefficients for the 14 domains range from 0.37 (unacceptable vocal habits) to 0.77 (use of medications), with a mean reliability coefficient of 0.57. In part, as a function of the less than optimal reliability of Part 2 of ABS1, the ABS2 contained only eight domains related to maladaptive behavior: (a) social behavior, (b) conformity, (c) trustworthiness, (d) stereotyped and hyperactive behavior, (e) sexual behavior, (f) self-abusive

Table 6.1 Reliability Coefficients for Adaptive Domains on ABS1 and ABS2

Domain	ABS1[a] interrater	ABS2[b] test–retest	ABS2[c] internal consistency
Independent functioning	0.92	0.99	0.98
Physical development	0.93	0.96	0.94
Economic development	0.85	0.98	0.90
Language development	0.87	0.96	0.96
Numbers and time	0.86	0.97	0.94
Domestic activity	0.91	0.99	0.95
Vocational activity	0.78	0.88	0.82
Self-direction	0.71	0.92	0.94
Responsibility	0.83	0.95	0.90
Socialization	0.77	0.88	0.91

[a]Mean Pearson product moment correlations using Fisher's Z transformation.
[b]Corrected reliability coefficient using Anastasi's[30] procedure for extracting error variance.
[c]Mean coefficient alpha averaged across age groups.

behavior, (g) social engagement, and (h) disturbing interpersonal behavior. Interrater reliability was much improved, with coefficients for the eight domains ranging from 0.95 (social behavior and conformity) to 0.99 (trustworthiness, self-abusive behavior, social engagement), with a mean reliability coefficient of 0.97.

Table 6.2 displays the reliability coefficients for each maladaptive domain in ABS1 and Table 6.3 displays the reliability coefficients for each maladaptive domain in ABS2.

Data regarding the validity of the 1974 and 1993 versions of the ABS were summarized by Meyers and colleagues,[23,25] and in the 1974 and 1993 ABS manuals.[14,21] Additionally, criterion validity was investigated by Salagaras and Nettelbeck,[31,32] who demonstrated the ABS's sensitivity to quantify individual differences in adaptive and maladaptive behavior among subgroups that varied with respect to seven variables: age, sex, estimated intellectual ability, etiology of ID, place of living, the presence or absence of any mobility handicap, and the use of prescription medications.

Adaptive behavior items on the ABS vary in type; some require a unitary response while others require respondents to select several responses. One type of item directs the rater to circle the statement that best describes the individual's abilities in the specific adaptive behavior among several choices, while the rater can circle multiple statements (i.e., all statements that apply) in the second type of item. Item scores are summed to provide subdomain scores, and subdomain scores are summed to provide domain scores. Percentile ranks are available for each domain, based upon an age-based comparison of an individual's score with the normative sample of 496 residents of institutions for people with ID.[14] (The ABS2 norming sample included 4103 individuals with ID residing with parents, in community-based small residences, or in large congregate care residential facilities.[21])

Table 6.2 Reliability Coefficients for Maladaptive Domains on ABS1

Domain	ABS1[a] interrater
Violent and destructive behavior	0.59
Antisocial behavior	0.68[b]
Rebellious behavior	0.55[b]
Untrustworthy behavior	0.69
Withdrawal	0.44
Stereotyped behavior and odd mannerisms	0.62[b]
Inappropriate interpersonal manners	0.47[b]
Unacceptable vocal habits	0.37[b]
Unacceptable or eccentric habits	0.57[b]
Self-abusive behavior	0.49[b]
Hyperactive tendencies	0.57
Sexually aberrant behavior	0.52[b]
Psychological disturbances	0.45[b]
Use of medications	0.77[b]

[a]Mean Pearson product moment correlations using Fisher's Z transformation.
[b]At least partially computed by phi coefficient.

Table 6.3 Reliability Coefficients for Maladaptive Domains on ABS2

Domain	ABS2[a] test–retest	ABS2[b] internal consistency
Social behavior	0.95	0.94
Conformity	0.95	0.91
Trustworthiness	0.99	0.88
Stereotyped and hyperactive behavior	0.96	0.86
Sexual behavior	0.98	0.83
Self-abusive behavior	0.99	0.81
Social engagement	0.99	0.84
Disturbing interpersonal behavior	0.97	0.90

[a]Corrected reliability coefficient using Anastasi's[30] procedure for extracting error variance.
[b]Mean coefficient alpha averaged across age groups.

Maladaptive behavior items on the ABS are all one type; the rater is directed to circle all statements that apply to the individual being evaluated in terms of the frequency of occurrence, occasionally or frequently. Item scores are again summed to provide subdomain scores, subdomain scores are summed to provide domain scores, and percentile ranks are available for each domain.

The ABS typically is administered through an interview with a correspondent familiar with the individual being assessed (i.e., "third-party assessment"), however alternate methods are available (see Fogelman and Nihira[14] for a complete description of administration options). Briefly, "first-person assessment" can be used when the rater is sufficiently familiar with the individual being evaluated that he or she can complete the form without referring to other sources for additional information. In the "interview method," the rater discusses the individual's behavioral competencies and maladaptive behaviors with a correspondent familiar with the individual being assessed. Subsequent to the interview, the rater independently completes the individual items on the ABS. This method of administration is not suggested for use in research when detailed information is required.[14]

Research Studies

ABS1 and Age-Related Changes in Adaptive Behavior: Cross-Sectional Studies

In 1983, Miniszek[33] reported the first use of the ABS1 to distinguish nine adults with DS over the age of 50 who were "seriously regressed" (i.e., demented) from six adults with DS over age 50 who exhibited no visible signs of dementia. All 15 adults with DS over age 50 also exhibited lower ABS1 domain scores compared with a small group with DS under the age of 50. In spite of this successful use of the ABS1 to classify dementia in this initial study, it was almost 10 years until the ABS1 was used in other efforts to describe functional and cognitive deterioration in adults with DS.[34,35] One such study examined ABS1 domain and total scores (i.e., Part 1 and Part 2), in adults with DS who ranged from 18 to over 60 years of age. Participants over 50 years of age manifested significantly poorer performance in most functional domains than did younger participants, with adults over age 60 exhibiting the lowest performance on all domains. There were no age-associated differences in ABS1 Part 2 domains (maladaptive behavior), with the exception of "use of medications," which was increased in the group of older adults.[34] A second study focused on language development measured by the ABS1 in adults with DS who had no major sensory impairments, and found that expressive language and comprehension performance was significantly reduced in older participants compared with younger participants, with the largest age-associated deficits found in comprehension skills.[35] Prasher,[36] using similar procedures also found age-associated differences in language development, however effects were equivalent in both the expressive language and the comprehension subdomains. This discrepancy may have been due to increased sensory function in the latter study, as Prasher directly assessed vision and hearing, while the earlier study was less precise.

Collacott[37] expanded these analyses to ascertain the effect of age of epilepsy onset (early <35 years of age versus late ≥35 years of age) on adaptive competence. Collacott suggested that epilepsy could serve as a surrogate indicator of DAD, as the onset of seizures is a well-known late-stage symptom.[38] Timing of epilepsy onset was significantly related to ABS1 adaptive scores, with individuals with late-onset epilepsy, compared with early-onset epilepsy, exhibiting poorer performance. Again, there were no significant differences in ABS1 Part 2 domains (maladaptive behavior) with the exception of "use of medications." Clearly, the ability to use the ABS1 to measure "age-associated differences" (i.e., differences in cohorts defined by age) in adaptive competence in adults with DS has been established, but the cross-sectional nature of the above studies limit their utility to demonstrate age-related declines (i.e., declines in the same cohort over time). Age-associated differences in adaptive competence may be due to aging and the presumed development of dementia, or they may be present simply because the sample members belong to different cohorts with different life experiences. These classic "cohort effects" arise because earlier life experiences can be important determinants of a population's characteristics in later life and may be related to the observed age-associated differences. For example, the better health care, nutrition, and education provided for people with DS born 30 years ago, varied widely with the neglect and maltreatment, in general, that people born with DS received 70 years ago. As a function of these effects, longitudinal studies of people born within the same cohort are necessary to clearly document decline over time.

ABS1 and Age-Related Changes in Adaptive Behavior: Longitudinal Studies

One of the first studies to use the ABS1 to measure longitudinal change in adaptive competence in adults with DS was conducted by Fenner et al.[39] Significant losses in functional abilities were exhibited only by one-third of the individuals over age

35, but the oldest participant was only 49 years old, and studies of older people should be necessary to answer the true extent of age-related adaptive decline to be found in adults with DS.

The ABS1 and Adaptive Behavior Change as a Surrogate Indicator of Dementia Classification

Zigman and colleagues examined the age-associated incidence of significant decline in adaptive behavior and the temporal pattern of decline in specific functional skill domains in 646 adults with ID with and without DS using the ABS1.[40,41] The standard error of measurement (SEM), a reflection of dispersion around an individual's true score with known statistical properties was computed, and significant decline in adaptive behavior was defined as a reduction of two SEMs in total ABS1 score over a 2-year period. Cumulative incidence of significant decline in total ABS1 score for adults with DS increased from 4% at age 50 to 67% by age 72, verifying that aging throughout the 50s and 60s is not uniformly pathologic by age 50; clearly a significant number of adults with DS are successfully surviving into their 60s and 70s.

While incidence rates for adults with DS reflect significant decline in total ABS1 score, and not dementia, these rates are not meaningfully different from published rates of classified dementia in DS.[42] Cumulative incidence of significant decline in total ABS1 score for adults with ID without DS increased from 2% at age 50 to 52% by age 88, fairly similar to prevalence rates of DAD in the typically developing population at that advanced age.[43,44]

The ABS1 was not designed as a metric of dementia; therefore, various domain and subdomain scores might be differentially sensitive to longitudinal changes in adaptive behavior. An a priori descriptive content analysis of the ABS1 resulted in the identification of 15 separate clusters of items. Changes over time were analyzed within each of the adaptive clusters only in participants who declined significantly in the overall adaptive functioning score. (An examination of nondecliners revealed that they were relatively stable over time in each of the 15 clusters.) Differences in the timing and magnitude of declines were evident, with relatively large and early declines in performance in care of clothing, dressing and undressing activities, domestic activities, and vocational activities.[41] Relatively early, but somewhat smaller declines in performance were seen in responsibility and socialization, economic activities, physical development, travel, and general independent functioning activities.[41] Proficiency in these skills also may be considered necessary to function competently in everyday activities of daily life outside the home. Clusters reflecting more basic activities of daily living skills declined slightly later. Larger declines were observed for self-direction, toilet use, numbers and time, and cleanliness.[41] Smaller declines were seen for comprehension and social language, appearance, eating, and expression.[41] These patterns also are consistent with the timing of dementia symptoms in typically developing adults. Functional declines are first noted in skills that are more complex with progression to the more basic and fundamental abilities. Not surprisingly, ability to eat, to understand spoken language, and to ambulate are among the last to be affected. These patterns are substantially consistent with previous reports describing the progression of dementia symptoms in adults with DS[45] and adults in the typically developing population.[46]

Changes in maladaptive behaviors in participants with significant changes in adaptive functioning were examined in a follow-up study using the ABS1 Part 2 maladaptive items.[40] Obnoxious behavior (e.g., lying, reacting poorly to frustration or criticism, demanding excessive attention, impudent attitude toward authority), lack of boundaries (e.g., takes others' property, disrespecting others' property), and overestimating one's own abilities were significantly elevated before the occurrence of subsequent significant adaptive decline and then decreased over time. These results suggest that elevated levels of these behaviors may anticipate significant regression in adaptive behavior and may provide caregivers with early indicators of concern. Changes that occurred concurrently with significant regression in adaptive behavior included withdrawn behavior and emotional instability (e.g., mood changes, poor emotional control). Caregivers also should take notice of these types of changes in "older" adults with ID, as they may be indicative of memory problems and disinhibition. Overall, these findings suggest that selected changes in specific areas of maladaptive behavior may be early signals of dementia in individuals with DS[47]; therefore, more research on these issues is certainly necessary. Data presented to this point clearly suggest that the ABS1 is sensitive to age-associated differences and age-related declines over time in adaptive competence; next, we will present the results of studies that measured ABS adaptive performance as a function of specific dementia classifications.

ABS and Dementia Classification: Cross-Sectional and Longitudinal Studies

Prasher and colleagues,[36,45,48–50] as part of a longitudinal investigation of aging and dementia in adults with DS, used the ABS1 to measure participants' adaptive competence and maladaptive behavior. Controlling for age, results from cross-sectional analyses demonstrated that participants with dementia had significantly lower total ABS1 scores than unaffected adults.[48] A subgroup of adults with DS without dementia who had no significant medical or psychiatric pathology still exhibited age-associated differences in adaptive competence, which may be demonstrating "normal" age-related changes in ability as opposed to dementia-related performance deficits; alternatively, they may just represent very early-stage DAD. Longitudinal changes in ABS1 scores in adults with DS were described in three additional studies reported by Prasher.[45,49,50] There were a number of methodological differences among the studies that included the sample characteristics, duration of follow-up, and the stage of dementia investigated. In one study, changes in adaptive competence were examined over a 2-year period ranging from 1-year before diagnosis of dementia to 1-year after diagnosis.[49] In the other two studies, changes in adaptive competence were examined as a function of dementia status (i.e., demented versus nondemented). Regardless of the methodological variations, essentially similar outcomes were obtained from all three studies. As adults with DS transition from nondemented to demented status, there are significant changes in adaptive competence and, as would be expected, the magnitude of these changes increases as dementia progresses. As noted previously, ABS1 Part 2 total scores were generally higher in participants with dementia compared to those without dementia.

Finally, two clinical trials examining the safety and efficiency of donepezil hydrochloride (Aricept) to slow the progression of dementia in adults with DS included the ABS1 as a measure of adaptive competence.[51,52] Results of these studies demonstrated the sensitivity and utility of the ABS1 as a metric for change even within a relatively restricted time.

ABS and Dementia: The Aging Research Program

A series of multidisciplinary longitudinal studies focusing on incidence, prevalence, risk factors and natural history of dementia and chronic health conditions in over 500 adults with ID with and without DS over the age of 45 have been conducted for over 10 years.[29,53] Dementia status has been assessed at 18-month intervals based upon measures of adaptive and cognitive functioning, a comprehensive review of all medications and clinical records, and a neurological examination to determine differential diagnoses for those participants suspected of having dementia. The Dementia Questionnaire for Mentally Retarded Persons[54,55] and Part I of the ABS has been used to measure adaptive competence and functional behavior, and the Reiss Screen for Maladaptive Behavior[56] to provide an overview of possible depression, psychosis, and maladaptive behavior that might mimic or be associated with dementia.

Cognitive abilities of participants have been described based upon eight direct assessment instruments. The Peabody Picture Vocabulary Test-Revised was used to provide a measure of receptive vocabulary.[57] Evaluation of mental status has been evaluated using three separate instruments: (a) a modified version of the Down Syndrome Mental Status Examination developed by Haxby,[58] (b) the IBRDD Mental Status Evaluation developed in our laboratories,[59] and (c) the Test for Severe Impairment.[60] The battery also includes an adaptation of the McCarthy verbal fluency test[61] and the Beery Visual Motor Integration test (long form),[62] the Block Design subtest of the WISC-R,[63] and an adaption of the Selective Reminding Test.[64] A full description of the instrument battery and its psychometric characteristics has been published elsewhere.[29,53] Dementia was classified in consensus conferences consistent with guidelines recommended by the Working Group for the Establishment of Criteria for the Diagnosis of Dementia in Individuals with Developmental Disability.[65,66] Each case was classified into one of the following categories: (a) nondemented, indicating that dementia was definitely not present, (b) questionable, indicating substantial uncertainty regarding dementia status, with some indications of mild functional and cognitive declines present, (c) possible dementia, indicating that some symptoms of dementia were present, but declines over time were not judged to be totally convincing, (d) definite dementia, indicating clear and convincing evidence of substantial decline over time, (e) uncertain with complications, indicating that criteria for definite dementia had been met, but that symptoms might be caused by some other substantial concern, usually a medical condition unrelated to a dementing disorder (e.g., depression, loss of vision, poorly resolved hip fracture, loss of social support network due to relocation), and (f) undeterminable, indicating that preexisting impairments were so severe that detection or interpretation of declines indicative of dementia were not possible.

Classification decisions inherently included a degree of subjective judgment that is difficult to quantify. This concern could be addressed by developing objective criteria for case classification. Of course, performance on any of these assessment measures is influenced by degree of developmental impairment as well as by dementia. Current recommendations for diagnosis of dementia recognize this by emphasizing the detection of decline from previous levels of performance.[65,66] However, this requires either that the process of diagnosis extends over substantial time intervals (often years) or that valid assessment of baseline abilities has been performed. The first of these requirements precludes rapid decision-making and intervention while the second is unlikely to occur. Therefore, our findings were examined in the hope of discovering classification criteria based upon a single assessment that considered level of preexisting impairment in addition to those that rely on detection of decline over extended periods of time.

Based upon the results described above, we developed an index that reflects the total score on ten subdomains of the ABS1 that were found to deteriorate relatively early in the progression of DAD (i.e., care of clothing, dressing and undressing, domestic activity, vocational activity, responsibility, socialization, economic activity, physical development, travel, and general independent functioning), hereafter called "the dementia sensitive index."[41] Performance on the dementia sensitive index was plotted as a function of intelligence quotient (IQ) for each dementia classification category. A function was generated that related performance on the dementia sensitive index to IQ and distinguished demented from nondemented individuals. This function was generated using data from the first data collection cycle and then verified with data collected in a subsequent cycle. These data are substantially less than independent, but they were useful to define a procedure to develop IQ-based dementia criteria. If the criterion score on the dementia sensitive index (total possible score 140) was defined by this equation $(10 + (1.5 * IQ))$, with a maximum score 75, the ability to correctly classify dementia in participants who were demented (i.e., sensitivity) was 0.9 and the ability to correctly classify participants who did not have dementia as nondemented (i.e., specificity) also was 0.9; for nondemented versus definite dementia cases.[67] We need to mention a few limitations of this metric: (a) these criteria were not useful with participants who had IQs less than 26, as IQ scores in that range are not considered reliable, (b) the estimates of sensitivity and specificity refer to distinctions between the two most extreme classification categories (nondemented and definite dementia), (c) these data classify dementia based on one instrument; optimally dementia status classifications should be based on measures of both adaptive and cognitive performance, and (d) these criteria need to be validated in an independent sample to be considered anything more than preliminary.

Summary

As adults age the risk for diseases such as dementia and DAD increase, especially so for people with DS who are prone to premature aging.[68] In the over 130 years since Fraser and Mitchell[11] first discussed skill loss in elderly adults with DS, there has been substantial progress in research probing the complex relationship between DS and AD. The origin of the ubiquitous AD-type pathology in adults with DS is related, at least in part, to the triplication of the gene for amyloid precursor protein, located on chromosome 21.[69,70] In the early 1980s, many researchers held the belief that all adults with DS who survived into their 40s and 50s would invariably develop clinical dementia. This dire prediction has proved untrue; many adults with DS are living successfully into their late 60s and even 70s.[71–74] Risk factors that may increase or decrease risk for DAD in adults with DS have been identified[75–82]; including some such as cholesterol level, statin use, and bioavailable estrogen, that may be amenable to alteration through medical intervention. Clinical trials should be conducted to test the safety and efficacy of these interventions; if they prove effective in delaying the onset or preventing DAD in adults with DS, this would result in an improved quality of life.

As this volume on neuropsychological measures of dementia in DS indicates, standard diagnostic methods used to evaluate individuals with suspected dementia in the general population are not appropriate for use with adults with DS, many of whom have never developed the specific cognitive and adaptive skills that are measured by these assessment instruments. The use of the ABS as a surrogate measure of dementia has met with considerable success. The other chapters in this volume demonstrate that there are multiple functional and neuropsychological measures that may be successfully used to classify dementia status in adults with DS. In fact, the emphasis of the ABS on functional behavior may result in dementia being diagnosed relatively late in the disease process. Optimally, a highly sensitive and specific assessment battery will eventually be developed that uses the most reliable and valid aspects of each instrument to classify dementia in DS at the earliest possible stage. Additionally, further research into the role of maladaptive behaviors in the identification of early signs of dementia also is warranted. There are a number of benefits of early diagnosis of dementia.[83] Treatments that are currently available, or are in the development stage will clearly work best during early stages of disease progression before severe neuronal loss has occurred. Additionally, there are a number of conditions that can cause a reversible- or pseudo-dementia that can be successfully managed given the correct diagnosis and therapeutic regimen (e.g., severe hypothyroidism, Cushing's syndrome, severe depression, adverse reactions to pharmaceuticals). Finally, if dementia is confirmed, coping strategies can be developed to minimize some of the behavioral and medical sequelae of the condition.

Currently, there are few if any reliable biomarkers of dementia in DS (or in the typically developing population). The development of biomarkers of dementia in DS could help validate the early diagnosis of DAD, and allow available treatments to be promptly initiated. While research regarding the DS/AD link has progressed substantially in the past 25 years, there still are many unanswered questions. We are confident that in the near future, valid biomarkers, more powerful clinical diagnostic methods, and effective treatments will be forthcoming, improving the quality of life for older adults with DS.

Acknowledgments Supported by NIH grants R01-AG014763, P01-HD35897, R01-HD37425, by the National Down Syndrome Society in collaboration with the NICHD, and by NYS through its Office of Mental Retardation and Developmental Disabilities.

References

1. Stratford B (1989) Down's Syndrome: Past, Present and Future. London: Penguin.
2. Stratford B (1982) Down's syndrome at the Court of Mantua. J Family Med: Matern Child Health 7:250–4.
3. Down JLH (1866) Observations on an ethnic classification of idiots. Lond Hosp Rep 3:259–62.
4. Lejeune J, Gautier M, and Turpin R (1959) Study of somatic chromosomes from 9 mongoloid children. CR Hebd Seances Acad Sci 248:1721–2.
5. Lejeune J, Gautier M, and Turpin R (1959) A study of somatic chromosomes in nine infants with mongolism. CR Acad Sci (Paris) 240:1026–7.
6. Centers for Disease Control and Prevention (CDC). (2006) Improved national prevalence estimates for 18 selected major birth defects—United States, 1999–2001. Morb Mortal Wkly Rep. 54:1301-1305.
7. American Psychiatric Association (1987) Diagnostic and Statistical Manual of Mental Disorders, 3rd edn., revised. Washington, DC: American Psychiatric Association.
8. Ackerman S (1992) The role of the brain in mental illness. In: Discovering the Brain. Washington, DC: National Academy Press, pp. 46–66.
9. Graeber MB, Kosel S, Egensperger R, et al. (1997) Rediscovery of the case described by Alois Alzheimer in 1911: Historical, histological and molecular genetic analysis. Neurogenetics 1:73–80.
10. Alzheimer A, Stelzmann RA, Schnitzlein HN, et al. (1995) An English translation of Alzheimer's 1907 paper, "Uber eine eigenartige Erkankung der Hirnrinde". Clin Anat 8:429–31.
11. Fraser J and Mitchell A (1876) Kalmuc idiocy: Report of a case with autopsy with notes on sixty-two cases. J Ment Sci 22:169–79.
12. Jervis GA (1948) Early senile dementia in mongoloid idiocy. Am J Psychiatry 105:102–6.
13. National Institute on Aging (2006) Aging Under the Microscope: A Biological Quest. National Institutes of Health 51.
14. Fogelman CJ and Nihira K (1975) AAMD Adaptive Behavior Scale: The American Association on Mental Deficiency, Washingdon DC.

15. Heber R (1961) A manual on terminology and classification in mental retardation. Am J Mental Deficiency (Monogr Suppl, 2nd Ed).
16. Grossman HE (1977) A Manual on Terminology and Classification in Mental Retardation, 3rd edn. Washington, DC: American Association on Mental Retardation.
17. Schalock RL (1999) The concept of adaptive behavior. In: Schalock RL, ed. Adaptive Behavior and Its Measurement: Implications for the Field of Mental Retardation. Washington, DC: American Association on Mental Retardation, pp. 1–5.
18. Leland H (1991) Adaptive behavior scales. In: Matson JL and Mulick JA, eds. Handbook of Mental Retardation, 2nd edn. New York: Pergamon Press, pp. 211–21.
19. Leland H, Shellhaas M, Nihira K, et al. (1967) Adaptive behavior: A new dimension in the qualification of the mentally retarded. Ment Retard Abstr 4:359–87.
20. Nihira K, Foster R, Shellhaas M, et-al. (1974) AAMD Adaptive Behavior Scale. Washington, DC: American Association on Mental Deficiency.
21. Nihira K, Leland H, and Lambert N (1993) American Association on Mental R. ABS-RC: 2, AAMR Adaptive Behavior Scale Residential and Community: PRO-ED.
22. Academy N (2002) The role of adaptive behavior assessment. In: Reschly DJ, Myers TG, and Hartel CR, eds. Mental Retardation: Determining Eligibility for Social Security Benefits. Washington, DC: National Academies Press, pp. 141–207.
23. Meyer CE, Nihira K, Zetlin A (1979) The measurement of adaptive behavior. In: Ellis NR, ed. Handbook of Mental Deficiency, Psychological Theory and Research, 2nd edn. Hillsdale, NJ: Lawrence Erlbaum Associates, pp. 431–81.
24. Isett RD and Spreat S (1979) Test-retest and interrater reliability of the AAMD adaptive behavior scale. Am J Ment Defic 84:93–5.
25. Spreat S (1980) The adaptive behavior scale: a study of criterion validity. Am J Ment Defic 85:61–8.
26. Knapp S and Salend SJ (1983) Adapting the Adaptive Behavior Scale. Ment Retard 21:63–7.
27. Malamud N (1972) Neuropathology of organic brain syndromes associated with aging. Aging Brain 63–87.
28. Lott IT and Head E (2005) Alzheimer disease and Down syndrome: factors in pathogenesis. Neurobiol Aging. 26:383–9.
29. Silverman W, Schupf N, Zigman W, et al. (2004). Dementia in adults with mental retardation: assessment at a single point in time. Am J Ment Retard 109:111–25.
30. Anastasi A (1988) Psychological Testing, 6th edn. New York: Macmillan.
31. Salagaras S and Nettelbeck T (1983) Adaptive behavior of mentally retarded adolescents attending school. Am J Ment Defic 88:57–68.
32. Salagaras S and Nettelbeck T (1984) Adaptive behavior of mentally retarded adults in work-preparation settings. Am J Ment Defic 88:437–41.
33. Miniszek NA (1983) Development of Alzheimer disease in Down syndrome individuals. Am J Ment Defic 87:377–85.
34. Collacott RA (1992) The effect of age and residential placement on adaptive behaviour of adults with Down's syndrome. Br J Psychiatry 161:675–9.
35. Cooper SA and Collacott RA (1995) The effect of age on language in people with Down's syndrome. J Intellect Disabil Res 39:197–200.
36. Prasher VP (1996) The effect of age on language in people with Down's syndrome. J Intellect Disabil Res 40:484–5.
37. Collacott RA (1993) Epilepsy, dementia and adaptive behaviour in Down's syndrome. J Intellect Disabil Res 37:153–60.
38. Amatniek JC, H ser WA, DelCastillo-Castaneda C, et al. (2006) Incidence and predictors of seizures in patients with Alzheimer's disease. Epilepsia 47:867–72.
39. Fenner ME, Hewitt KE, and Torpy DM (1987) Down's syndrome: Intellectual and behavioural functioning during adulthood. J Ment Defic Res 31:241–9.
40. Urv TK, Zigman WB, and Silverman W (2003) Maladaptive behaviors related to adaptive decline in aging adults with mental retardation. Am J Ment Retard 108:327–39.

41. Zigman WB, Schupf N, Urv T, et al. (2002) Incidence and temporal patterns of adaptive behavior change in adults with mental retardation. Am J Ment Retard 107:161–74.
42. Visser FE, Aldenkamp AP, van Huffelen AC, et al. (1997) Prospective study of the prevalence of Alzheimer-type dementia in institutionalized individuals with Down syndrome. Am J Ment Retard 101:400–12.
43. Henderson S (1998) Epidemiology of dementia. Ann Med Intern (Paris) 149:181–6.
44. Borjesson-Hanson A, Edin E, Gislason T, et al. (2004) The prevalence of dementia in 95 year olds. Neurology 28(63):2436–8.
45. Prasher VP, Chung MC, and Haque MS (1998) Longitudinal changes in adaptive behavior in adults with Down syndrome: Interim findings from a longitudinal study. Am J Ment Retard 103:40–6.
46. Perneczky R, Pohl C, Sorg C, et al. (2006) Impairment of activities of daily living requiring memory or complex reasoning as part of the MCI syndrome. Int J Geriatr Psychiatry 21:158–62.
47. Ball SL, Holland AJ, Hon J, et al. (2006) Personality and behaviour changes mark the early stages of Alzheimer's disease in adults with Down's syndrome: Findings from a prospective population-based study. Int J Geriatr Psychiatry 21:661–73.
48. Prasher VP and Chung MC (1996) Causes of age-related decline in adaptive behavior of adults with Down syndrome: Differential diagnoses of dementia. Am J Ment Retard 101:175–83.
49. Prasher VP (1996) Is there a prodromal phase to Alzheimer's dementia in adults with Down syndrome? Br J Develop Disabil 42:192–7.
50. Prasher VP, Krishnan DJ, Clarke DJ, et al. (1994) The assessment of dementia in people with Down syndrome: Changes in adaptive behaviour. Br J Dev Disabil XL:120–30.
51. Prasher VP, Adams C, and Holder R (2003) Long term safety and efficacy of donepezil in the treatment of dementia in Alzheimer's disease in adults with Down syndrome: Open label study. Int J Geriatr Psychiatry 18:549–51.
52. Prasher VP, Huxley A, and Haque MS (2002) A 24-week, double-blind, placebo-controlled trial of donepezil in patients with Down syndrome and Alzheimer's disease—pilot study. Int J Geriatr Psychiatry 17:270–8.
53. Zigman WB, Schupf N, Devenny DA, et al. (2004) Incidence and prevalence of dementia in elderly adults with mental retardation without Down syndrome. Am J Ment Retard 109:126–41.
54. Evenhuis HM (1996) Further evaluation of the Dementia Questionnaire for Persons with Mental Retardation (DMR). J Intellect Disabil Res 40:369–73.
55. Evenhuis HM (1992) Evaluation of a screening instrument for dementia in ageing mentally retarded persons. J Intellect Disabil Res 36:337–47.
56. Reiss S and Valenti-Hein D (1994) Development of a psychopathology rating scale for children with mental retardation. J Consult Clin Psychol 62:28–33.
57. Dunn L and Dunn L (1981) Peabody Picture Vocabulary Test-Revised. Circle Pines, MN: American Guidance Service.
58. Haxby JV (1989) Neuropsychological evaluation of adults with Down's syndrome: Patterns of selective impairment in non-demented old adults. J Ment Defic Res 33:193–210.
59. Wisniewski K and Hill A, eds (1985) Clinical Aspects of Dementia in Mental Retardation and Developmental Disabilities. Baltimore, MD: Brookes.
60. Albert M and Cohen C (1992) The Test for Severe Impairment: An instrument for the assessment of patients with severe cognitive dysfunction. J Am Geriatr Soc 40:449–53.
61. McCarthy D (1972) Scales of Children's Abilities. San Antonio, TX: Psychological Corporation.
62. Beery K and Bukenia N (1989) Developmental Test of Visual-Motor Integration. Cleveland, OH: Modern Curriculum Press.
63. Wechsler D (1974) Wechsler Intelligence Scale for Children-Revised. New York, NY: Psychological Corporation.
64. Buschke H (1973) Selective reminding for analysis of memory and learning. J Verbal Learn Verbal Behav 12:543–50.

65. Aylward EH, Burt DB, Thorpe LU, et al. (1997) Diagnosis of dementia in individuals with intellectual disability. J Intellect Disabil Res 41:152–64.
66. Burt DB and Aylward EH (2000) Test battery for the diagnosis of dementia in individuals with intellectual disability. Working Group for the Establishment of Criteria for the Diagnosis of Dementia in Individuals with Intellectual Disability. J Intellect Disabil Res 44:175–80.
67. Silverman W, Devenny DA, Krinsky-McHale SJ, et al. (2006) Aging, dementia and cognitive decline in adults with Down syndrome. In: 39th Annual Gatlinburg Conference on Research and Theory in Intellectual and Developmental Disabilities, San Diego.
68. Lott IT (1982) Down's syndrome, aging, and Alzheimer's disease: A clinical review. Ann N Y Acad Sci 396:15–27.
69. Goldgaber D, Lerman MI, McBride WO, et al. (1987) Isolation, characterization, and chromosomal localization of human brain cDNA clones coding for the precursor of the amyloid of brain in Alzheimer's disease, Down's syndrome and aging. J Neural Transm Suppl 24:23–8.
70. Prasher VP, Farrer MJ, Kessling AM, et al. (1998) Molecular mapping of Alzheimer-type dementia in Down's syndrome. Ann Neurol 43:380–3.
71. Lai F and Williams RS (1989) A prospective study of Alzheimer disease in Down syndrome. Arch Neurol 46:849–53.
72. Zigman WB, Schupf N, Sersen E, et al. (1996) Prevalence of dementia in adults with and without Down syndrome. Am J Ment Retard 100:403–12.
73. Holland AJ, Hon J, Huppert FA, et al. (1998) Population-based study of the prevalence and presentation of dementia in adults with Down's syndrome. Br J Psychiatry 172:493–8.
74. Zigman W, Jenkins E, Mehta P, et al. (2000) Alzheimer's disease, survival, and genetics in the "oldest old" with Down syndrome. In: Down Syndrome Research Foundation (Canada)/National Down Syndrome Society (US) New Directions in Down Syndrome Research Conference, Toronto, Canada.
75. Jackson CV, Holland AJ, Williams CA, et al. (1988) Vitamin E and Alzheimer's disease in subjects with Down's syndrome. J Ment Defic Res 32:479–84.
76. Schupf N, Kapell D, Lee JH, et al. (1996) Onset of dementia is associated with apolipoprotein E epsilon4 in Down's syndrome. Ann Neurol 40:799–801.
77. Cosgrave M, Tyrrell J, Dreja H, et al. (1996) Lower frequency of apolipoprotein E4 allele in an "elderly" Down's syndrome population. Biol Psychiatry 15:811–3.
78. Folin M, Baiguera S, Conconi MT, et al. (2003) The impact of risk factors of Alzheimer's disease in the Down syndrome. Int J Mol Med 11:267–70.
79. Schupf N, Pang D, Patel BN, et al. (2003) Onset of dementia is associated with age at menopause in women with Down's syndrome. Ann Neurol 54:433–8.
80. Jenkins EC, Velinov MT, Ye L, et al. (2005) Telomere shortening in T lymphocytes of older individuals with Down syndrome and dementia. Neurobiol Aging. Jul 18, 27:941–945.
81. Schupf N, Winsten S, Patel B, et al. (2006) Bioavailable estradiol and age at onset of Alzheimer's disease in postmenopausal women with Down syndrome. Neurosci Lett 406:298–302.
82. Zigman WB, Schupf N, Jenkins EC, et al. (2007) Cholesterol level, statin use and Alzheimer's disease in adults with Down syndrome. Neurosci Lett 11:279–84.
83. National Institute on Aging (2003) Alzheimer's Disease: Unraveling the Mystery. U.S. Department of Human Services, National Institutes of Health.

Chapter 7
The Cambridge Examination for Mental Disorders of Older People with Down's Syndrome and Others with Intellectual Disabilities (CAMDEX-DS)

A.J. Holland and S.L. Ball

Background

The Cambridge Examination for Mental Disorders of Older People with Down's Syndrome and Others with Intellectual Disabilities (CAMDEX-DS) is a diagnostic assessment schedule that was developed in response to an identified need for valid and reliable methods for the assessment and diagnosis of dementia in people with intellectual disability (ID). While the increased risk of dementia in people with Down syndrome (DS) in particular means that the schedule is especially valuable for use in this population, it can also been used when dementia is suspected in those with developmentally acquired ID for reasons other than that of DS. Accurate and consistent diagnosis is essential for both clinical practice and research and will be increasingly important as more effective treatments become available and as the prevalence of dementia increases in association with the improved life expectancy of people with DS.

Rationale for the Development of the CAMDEX-DS

The principal aims for the development of this assessment were [1] to incorporate in a single schedule all the information necessary to enable an accurate clinical diagnosis of dementia in people with ID, in the context of clinical practice or research, [2] to provide a structured framework for collecting information on the key features of the dementias and of other physical and psychiatric disorders of later life, in order to aid the differential diagnosis of any observed decline, with reference to standard operational diagnostic criteria, and [3] to provide a means for monitoring progress and informing social, psychological, and medical interventions.

While the diagnosis of dementia is complicated by the presence of preexisting ID, the principle that such a diagnosis requires evidence of a progressive deterioration in memory, in a number of other cognitive domains and in daily living skills, is the same regardless of whether an individual has ID. In the general population, a diagnosis of

V.P. Prasher (ed.), *Neuropsychological Assessments of Dementia in Down Syndrome and Intellectual Disabilities*,
DOI: 10.1007/978-1-84800-249-4_7, © Springer Science+Business Media, LLC 2009

dementia is reached on the basis of informant-based and objective evidence of progressive deterioration in a person's cognitive abilities and functional skills, the operational definitions generally accepted being those outlined in the *Diagnostic and Statistical Manual of Mental Disorders* (DSM-IV)[2] and the *International Classification of Diseases* (ICD-10).[3] Our approach in developing a diagnostic assessment for use with people with ID has been to model it very closely on an assessment schedule that is widely used as an aid to the diagnostic process in the general population; the revised version of the *Cambridge Examination for Mental Disorders of the Elderly* (CAMDEX-R).[4]

Like the original schedule, the CAMDEX-DS has been designed to be administered in community settings by mental health professionals (as part of the diagnostic process), or to be used to formalize diagnosis in the context of a research study and is designed to provide structure and support for good clinical and/or research practice. Arriving at a diagnosis of dementia requires a full evaluation and the elimination of other possible illnesses or disorders that might present in a similar manner to that of dementia. These disorders may be treatable and have a very different prognosis to that of dementia. Research studies[6] into the relationship between DS and dementia also require a similar level of diagnostic rigor. The CAMDEX-DS is not a substitute for proper clinical assessment when dementia is suspected, but rather it is an aid to the diagnostic process, designed for use by experienced clinicians and for informed clinical researchers. The diagnosis of dementia, or of other mental or physical disorders, though aided and supported by this framework, remains a judgment based on a clinical history, direct cognitive, mental state and physical assessments, and findings from appropriate investigations. In this respect, the CAMDEX-DS differs in both its aim and format from existing observer-rated scales that have been developed specifically for diagnosing dementia of the Alzheimer's type (DAT) (c.f., dementia in Alzheimer's disease (DAD) in people with ID that work on the principle of using a cutoff score to determine whether or not an individual has dementia. Such scales can be viewed as screening tools rather than aids to the process of making a clinical diagnosis.

Development and Use of the CAMDEX in the General Elderly Population

The CAMDEX was originally developed in 1986 as a standardized instrument for the diagnosis of mental disorder in the elderly general population, with particular reference to the early detection of dementia.[5] It was subsequently published by Cambridge University Press[6] and a revised version was published in 1998.[4] The schedule includes an informant interview, an interview with the participant, an objective examination of cognitive function (Cambridge Cognitive Examination, CAMCOG), a standardized schedule for recording observations, and a physical examination and information on laboratory investigations.

The informant interview provides a means for collecting information in a structured manner about those areas of function that are likely to change with the onset of dementia or of any other mental disorder. It includes several questions about the informant's observations on each of the following: the person's memory, general mental and intellectual functioning, judgment, general performance, specific higher cortical functions and personality, as well as the presence or absence of specific symptoms and relevant medical and family history.

The validity and reliability of the CAMDEX informant interview for use in the general elderly population has been shown to be good. For example, reported changes in memory and mental functioning from the informant interview highly correlated with objectively measured decline.[7] On measures of interrater reliability in the general population the correlation between total scores obtained by the two raters has been found to be high ($r = 0.90$, $p < 0.001$) as has the level of agreement on individual items (median phi coefficient = 0.91, range = 1.0–0.56).[5]

The CAMCOG is a concise neuropsychological test battery for the assessment of cognitive impairment in elderly people, which forms part of the CAMDEX schedule.[6] The CAMCOG was designed to assist in the diagnosis of dementia. It covers the broad range of cognitive functions that are known to decline in dementia,[8] and includes items that assess all those areas of decline specified in operational diagnostic criteria, such as DSM-IV[2] and ICD-10.[3] The CAMCOG enables the examination of profiles of cognitive performance, through the derivation of subscale scores, and permits the measurement of cognitive decline across a wide range of levels of premorbid ability, by covering a wide range of item difficulty. The CAMCOG items are divided into seven subscales, covering the following areas of cognitive function: orientation, language, memory, praxis, attention/calculation, abstract thinking, and perception. A number of these broad areas are subdivided into more specific domains. Language, for example, is divided into comprehension and expression, and memory items include those to assess remote and recent memory, intentional and incidental learning, and recall and recognition measures of retrieval. A revised version of the CAMCOG (CAMCOG-R) incorporated alternative remote memory questions for younger participants and also included two additional items to assess executive function (EF) in more detail: ideational fluency and visual reasoning. These items were not included in the CAMCOG-R total score, but enabled the calculation of a separate EFs score.

The CAMCOG has been shown to be reliable when used in the general population.[9] Total CAMCOG score has excellent internal reliability (Cochran's alpha 0.82, 0.89 in different samples) and test–retest reliability (Pearson correlation 0.86) and the reliability of individual subscales is acceptable (Pearson test–retest reliability 0.46–0.80). The validity of the CAMCOG has also been confirmed in a number of studies. The CAMCOG total score and each subscale score have been found to differ significantly between individuals with and without dementia, in an elderly population sample.[9,10] The CAMCOG has been used in many published studies, both clinical[11,12] and population based.[13–16] Many neuropsychological,[17,18] neuropathological,[19,20] and neuroimaging studies[21,22] have utilized the CAMCOG for the assessment of elderly demented and nondemented participants in the general population.

Modification of the CAMDEX Schedule for Use with Adults with Down Syndrome

The CAMDEX-DS differs from the CAMDEX-R on which it is based, by placing a much greater emphasis on the informant interview as the key to an accurate diagnosis. It acknowledges that a combination of developmentally acquired ID and the possible development of dementia may make it difficult to obtain a reliable history from the affected person him/herself. This is particularly the case for those with preexisting severe or profound ID. In addition, in order to take into account the substantial variation in the level of cognitive and functional ability across individuals with preexisting ID, the informant interview included in the CAMDEX-DS schedule has been modified, to place greater importance on establishing decline from the individuals best level of functioning. While a direct cognitive assessment is still included in the CAMDEX-DS, we have suggested that testing cognitive ability at a single point in time does little to aid differential diagnosis. In the non-ID population deterioration can generally be inferred from the observation of a low level of performance relative to population norms. However, for individuals with an ID, it is particularly important to establish change explicitly, since cognitive impairment may be due to the underlying ID, rather than to the development of dementia. The cognitive assessment included in the CAMDEX-DS (which retains the same structure as the original CAMCOG, but has been modified to make it more suitable for use with people with ID) is intended to form a useful adjunct to the diagnostic process, when used to detect change over time through repeated assessment.

Modification of the CAMDEX Informant Interview

The modification of the CAMDEX informant interview took into account the fact that the cognitive and functional abilities affected by dementia may be impaired prior to the onset of dementia, due to the person's preexisting ID. Questions elucidating the presence of a particular problem (e.g., "Does he or she have difficulty in remembering recent events?") are followed up with questions to determine whether this is a deterioration in the individual's behavior or functioning, or whether it has always been a problem (i.e., "Is this a deterioration?"). There must be evidence of deterioration in that particular function (e.g., memory), as observed by the informant, if, when rating the information against operational diagnostic criteria, it is to be scored as being present as a symptom of dementia.

While the majority of the questions included in the CAMDEX-DS informant interview are based on those included in CAMDEX-R, there has been some restructuring of the schedule, in terms of section headings and the questions included within each section, to increase the ease with which the answers can be related directly to diagnostic criteria. Questions from Part I and II of the CAMDEX-R informant interview "Items concerned with history of present difficulty" and "Questions pertaining to the subject's past history" have been redistributed into three parts "Cognitive and Functional Decline" (which includes questions relevant to the identification of features of dementia), "Current Mental Health," and "Current Physical Health" (which include questions on other potential explanations for cognitive and functional deterioration, e.g., depression, thyroid disorder, sensory impairment or serious illness). The CAMDEX-DS informant interview begins with additional questions on "Patient/Participant's Best Level of Functioning," including questions on education and employment, basic skills (such as speech, language comprehension, reading, etc.) and independent living skills (such as dressing, food preparation, housework, etc.) in order to provide an overview of the individual's level of ability prior to the onset of any decline.

The "Cognitive and Functional Decline" part of the CAMDEX-DS informant interview begins with a section on "Everyday Skills," which covers changes in usual daytime activities, e.g., employment or day-center, preparation of food and drinks, housework, shopping (incorporating questions from various sections of the CAMDEX-R, including the direct "Interview with the patient/subject," with additional questions based on items from the Activities of Daily Living Scale,[23] and an explicit question on "difficulties at work, college or day-center"). The next section covers "Memory and Orientation" and includes all the questions from the "Memory" section of the CAMDEX-R (on recent memory/forgetfulness and orientation to place) with the addition of questions on remote memory and orientation in time (see Appendix 5 for example of CAMDEX-DS questions). The section on "Other Cognitive Skills" covers general mental functioning, language, perception, praxis and EFs and incorporates questions from the "General Mental Functioning" section of the CAMDEX-R informant interview, with additional questions on the following: slowness of thought, deterioration in reading/writing ability, language comprehension, ability to carry out familiar complex tasks, and day-to-day problem solving. These additional questions relate directly to operational diagnostic criteria regarding decline in cognitive functions other than memory. The final section covers "Personality, Behavior, and Self-Care," and incorporates questions from the "Personality," section of the CAMDEX-R informant interview, with selected questions from the "General Mental Functioning" and "Everyday Activities" sections. Additional questions on loss of personality and emotional flatness are included to relate specifically to CAMDEX criteria for dementia.

Modification of the CAMCOG

The majority of the items included in CAMCOG-DS are taken directly from the CAMCOG and the structure of the assessment remains the same. For those items that were found to be too difficult for many people with ID, the item was modified if possible, or otherwise replaced with an easier item assessing the same area of function. The revised version of the CAMCOG (CAMCOG-R)[4] provisionally included additional tests of EF that could be used to calculate a separate EF score. These were not included in CAMCOG-DS due to their high level of difficulty.

However, there are two measures included in CAMCOG-DS that can be regarded as EF measures: verbal fluency and similarities. The modifications made to the CAMCOG-DS mean that people with ID are more likely to score above the floor of the individual domains of this test (and on the test overall) than on the original CAMCOG, thereby enabling any loss of function to be determined over time.

The items that were omitted from the CAMCOG-DS because they were too difficult for the majority of individuals who took part in our ongoing study of aging and dementia in people with DS were: orientation items on date, season, county, two nearby streets, and floor of the building, comprehension items requiring a verbal yes/no response, two items on retrieval of recent information ("Who is likely to be the next King or Queen?" and "What has been in the news in the past week or two?"), the most difficult expression definition item ("What is an opinion?"), calculation items requiring the addition of two coins of different values and calculating required change and the most difficult abstract thinking item ("In what way are a plant and animal alike?"). A number of items were included in the CAMCOG-R assessment that did not contribute to the total CAMCOG-R score (but enabled the calculation of scores for alternative scales). These items were also omitted: "Write a complete sentence," "ideational praxis," "visual reasoning," "passage of time."

Minor modifications were made to a number of items, either by way of simplification or adjustments to the scoring. For the orientation questions that were retained, the scoring was changed so that 2 points were awarded if the correct answer was given without prompting and 1 point if the answer was given after a multiple choice prompt. For the comprehension questions requiring a motor response, credit was given for partially correct responses, e.g., for the item "touch your right ear with your left hand," 2 points are awarded for the correct response, and 1 point if partially correct (i.e., touches ear but with wrong hand). Some simplification was also made to the sentence construction for two of the motor response items; "before looking at the ceiling please look at the floor" was simplified to "please look at the ceiling and then look at the floor" and "tap each shoulder twice with two fingers keeping your eyes shut" was shortened to "please tap each shoulder twice with two fingers." For the tasks requiring the naming, recognition and recall of six pictures, the task structure remains unchanged but the pictures have been updated. The typewriter has been replaced with a computer and the barometer has been replaced with clock (since very few participants were able to name this item).

The retrieval of remote memories section was one that individuals with DS found particularly difficult. Little success was achieved on these questions, even using those modified for use with a younger population from the CAMCOG-R. Questions such as "Who led the Germans in the second world war?", "When did the Second World War begin?," and "Which American president was shot it Texas?" were omitted and replaced with two questions more likely to be familiar to our target population, "Who was John Lennon?" and "Which princess died in a car crash in Paris?" The scoring system was also modified so that 2 points are awarded if the correct answer is given without a prompt and 1 point is awarded if a clue is given (i.e., he was in a famous pop group, she was married to Prince Charles). The retrieval of recent information items also caused some difficulty and only the two easiest items were retained, "What is the name of the present king or queen?" and "What is the name of the prime minister?" Again the scoring was modified, as for the remote memory questions. The remembering a name and address item was included in a modified form. The majority of participants had been unable to write down the name and address on an envelope as required in the original item, so instead the participants are shown a picture of a man, and told his name and address, asked to repeat it and told to remember it for later. At a later point, after an intervening task, the participants is shown the picture of the man again and asked "What was this man's name?" and "What was his address?" In the copying and drawing section, the 3-D house was retained, but the scoring was altered so that points were awarded for each component successfully completed—up to a maximum of 3 points.

A number of difficult items were replaced with similar but easier items included in the Severe Impairment Battery,[24] a test that was developed to assess decline in people with severe dementia that has been shown to be valid for use with people with DS.[25] The expression repetition item "no ifs and/or buts" was replaced with "People Spend Money." Two attention items, "count backwards from 20" and "serial sevens" (in which the participant had to start at 100 and repeatedly subtract 7 until told to stop) were replaced with simpler items, counting to 20, counting the number of fingers held up by the Examiner and a forward digit span task (requiring the repetition of digit strings of between 1 and 5 digits in length). The most difficult reading comprehension item "If you are older than 50 put your hands behind your head" was replaced with the simpler "Give me your hand." For the copying and drawing task the linked hexagons and spiral were replaced with a simple square and circle.

Validity and Reliability of the CAMDEX-DS

Validity and Reliability of the CAMDEX-DS Informant Interview as an Aid to Dementia Diagnosis

The validity and reliability of the modified CAMDEX informant interview for use in the diagnosis of DAT in people with DS were examined using data from a population-based study.[26] The concurrent validity of the instrument was found to be good. Diagnoses based on the CAMDEX informant interview were validated against objective evidence of decline in cognitive functioning. Decline was measured over a period of approximately 6 years prior to diagnosis, using the CAMCOG neuropsychological test battery. Diagnostic category was found to discriminate well between those who had previously shown decline of greater than the mean change + 1 SD in CAMCOG score and those who had not. Those with a diagnosis of DAT were at least eight times more likely to have shown decline in neuropsychological test performance over the preceding 6 years, than those without a diagnosis of DA. Point estimates of sensitivity and specificity for the CAMDEX informant interview were shown to be high (0.88 and 0.94, respectively) and comparable with the levels found for the Dementia Questionnaire for Mentally Retarded Persons (DMR) and Dementia Scale for Down Syndrome (DSDS).[27] However, the small number of participants with DAT in the study, and resulting width of the 95% confidence interval for the sensitivity score, mean that these should be interpreted with caution.

The predictive validity of informant interview-based diagnoses was also shown to be good. None of the DAT diagnoses made at the baseline assessment were reversed at follow up approximately 6 years later. Those with a diagnosis of DAT at baseline were at least six times more likely to be diagnosed with DAT (or have died following DAT) at follow up than those without a baseline diagnosis of DAT. The follow-up diagnoses were all made blind to knowledge of previous diagnoses, thus ruling out potential bias. Although numbers were too small for the authors to draw any firm conclusions, the study also provided some support for the accuracy of the CAMDEX in predicting cognitive decline.

Only three participants with DAT at baseline were able to participate in the neuropsychological assessment at follow up. However, all three showed a decline of more than the mean + 1 SD on the CAMCOG, and this degree of decline was found to be significantly more likely to occur in those with DAT at baseline than in those without ($p < 0.005$, Fisher's exact). A number of participants were shown to have developed DAT in the 6-year period between baseline and follow-up assessment. These also showed decline in neuropsychological test performance.

Interrater reliability was also examined and shown to be very good. Data were reported for a subset of 20 people with DS, four of whom had DAT. The responses of the informants were rated simultaneously and independently by a psychiatrist, who conducted the informant interview, and a psychologist (the author) who observed. For each participant the ratings were compared for all items in the interview. Agreement between raters was shown to be excellent, with 91% of items falling within the "near perfect" range (Kappa > 0.8) and all items showing an agreement of Kappa > 0.6 (substantial), as defined by Landis and Koch.[28]

Although the results of the study are highly supportive of the validity of the informant interview, the relatively small number of participants with DAT in the study limits both the strength of the conclusions that can be drawn and the degree to which validity measures can be compared with those of other methods of diagnosis. However, the CAMDEX informant interview is currently the only tool for the assessment of DAT in DS to have been evaluated with regard to predictive validity and to use internationally agreed criteria to make DAT diagnoses. This study is also the first in this field to have demonstrated validity as measured against objective evidence of neuropsychological decline (a much stronger comparison than clinician's diagnosis).

Psychometric Properties of the CAMCOG-DS

As discussed above, the CAMCOG-DS is included in the CAMDEX-DS schedule to provide additional information that is useful in the diagnosis of dementia in people with DS. Findings have been published regarding the ability of the

CAMCOG to differentiate cross-sectionally between older and younger participants with DS.[29] Scores on the CAMCOG have been found to be well distributed, with only eight participants (11%) scoring zero on the test. This contrasted favorably with performance on the Mini-Mental State Examination[30] where there was a narrower range of scores and a higher percentage scoring zero. There was a significant difference in cognitive performance between younger (30–44 years) and older (45+ years) participants on the total CAMCOG score and on six out of the seven CAMCOG subscales. The study found that the CAMCOG, with minor modifications was a useful test to assess those areas of cognitive function known to decline with dementia. Apart from those with preexisting severe ID, severe sensory impairments and/or already advanced dementia, people with DS were able to score above the floor of the test.

In addition, participants with a diagnosis of dementia have been shown to decline to a greater degree on the CAMCOG than those without. The CAMCOG-DS included in the published CAMDEX-DS schedule has been further modified, to ensure that the majority of people with DS are able to score above the floor of the tests, thus better enabling the detection of cognitive decline. Validity not established for further modified CAMCOG-DS. Items with floor effects removed and replaced with easier items—should have the effect of making the measure more sensitive to the presence of dementia.

It should be noted however, that the CAMCOG-DS has limited diagnostic value at a single assessment, as without a baseline measure, it is not possible to determine the extent to which poor cognitive function is a consequence of a person's ID, any developing dementia, or any other disorder that might affect cognitive ability. However, the charting of decline in cognitive test scores over time provides a useful adjunct to the diagnostic process and may be constructive in informing support strategies.

Using the CAMDEX-DS

Administration of the Assessment Schedule

As outlined above, the CAMDEX-DS assessment schedule comprises an informant interview and a direct assessment of the patient/participant.

The CAMDEX-DS informant interview is a structured interview, comprising the following four parts: (1) best level of functioning, (2) cognitive and functional decline, (3) current mental health, and (4) current physical health. It has been designed to be carried out in the absence of the patient/participant, with a relative or carer who knows him/her well. The interview should be face-to-face whenever possible, but satisfactory information can be obtained from telephone interviews. The interview consists of approximately 150 questions in total and takes around 40 min to complete. Its aim is to facilitate the systematic collection of information about the presenting symptoms and clinical history. As illustrated in Fig. 7.1, in the section of the interview focused on cognitive and functional decline, each question is in two parts, the first establishing whether there is a problem in a particular area (e.g., recent memory) and the second establishing whether this is a deterioration.

Due to the particular emphasis placed on the importance of observed change from the individual's baseline level of functioning, the interview should be carried out with an informant who has known the person with DS well, for at least 6 months. For each question, answers are coded as follows: "no" = 0, "don't know" = 8, and "not applicable" = 9. Positive responses are coded either as 1 for "yes" or are graded in terms of severity, e.g., for questions regarding whether there is a deterioration, "slight deterioration" is coded as 1 and "great deterioration" is coded as 2. These codes are intended to aid the recording and storage of data. It should be noted however, that they are not intended to contribute toward a total score. Diagnosis should be based on the rating of responses against diagnostic criteria as described below.

The section of the CAMDEX-DS schedule, that is, completed directly with the patient/participant him/herself, includes both subjective report and objective measurement of decline in function associated with dementia or other mental or physical disorders and comprises the following three parts: (1) clinical interview, (2) cognitive assessment, and (3) interviewer observations. The clinical interview is a brief structured interview with the patient/participant, consisting of 13 questions, covering basic background information, current mental state, and additional information regarding presenting symptoms of dementia. Interviewer observations regarding present mental state, appearance, and demeanor are recorded using a standardized schedule. For both, answers are coded as for the informant interview and information is intended to provide additional support to carer observations when rating against diagnostic criteria for dementia.

The cognitive assessment (CAMCOG-DS) has been modified from the original CAMCOG, as described above, with the aim of assessing all the cognitive deficits specified in operational diagnostic criteria, i.e., memory impairment, aphasia, apraxia, agnosia, and disturbance in thinking (EF), using tasks that are suitable for use with people with a preexisting ID. Items within each cognitive domain are graded in difficulty to permit assessment within the full range of cognitive ability. The assessment covers the following domains: orientation, language (comprehension and expression), memory (new learning, remote, and recent), attention, praxis (drawing of complex figures and ability to carry out complex tasks), abstract thinking, and perception, all of which are known to decline with dementia. CAMCOG-DS provides subscale scores for hypothetically dissociable functions, as well as a total score with a maximum of 109. Each item contributes between 1 and 6 points to

Q No.	Does he/she have difficulties with ...?	Yes	1	→	Is this a deterioration?	Yes	→	Slight deterioration	1
								Great deterioration	2
		No	0			No	0		
		DK	8			DK	8		
	(a)	N/A	9	(b)		N/A	9		

Fig. 7.1 Example question

the relevant subscale and to the total score. Comparison of scores over assessments repeated at intervals of 6 months or more is intended to supplement subjective information regarding cognitive deterioration when making a diagnosis.

Diagnostic Process

In addition to the assessment schedule described above, the CAMDEX-DS pack also includes guidance regarding how to use the information gained through this assessment to inform the clinical diagnosis of dementia. The process of diagnosis essentially has three stages, as listed below, each of which is covered by one or more of the sections in the CAMDEX-DS:

1. A systematic history from the person him/herself and from an informant who has known that person over time, to establish the onset and course of the presenting problem (CAMDEX-DS patient and informant interviews).
2. A physical and mental state examination and cognitive assessments (CAMCOG-DS) and other investigations to enable the evaluation of present functioning and the identification of other possible causes of decline. The medical investigations should be guided by the clinical picture but invariably include investigations of a person's basic physical state (e.g., kidney and liver function and the presence or not of anemia) and specific tests, such as measures of thyroid function, or specialist assessment of hearing and/or vision. Where the clinical picture is unusual or the diagnosis is in doubt a computerized tomography (CT) or magnetic resonance imaging (MRI) brain scan may be indicated.
3. A detailed formulation and the evaluation of findings against known criteria for dementia and for other physical and mental disorders in order to arrive at a definitive diagnosis. For people with DS, three particular disorders are common and their presentation may mimic that of dementia as well as coexist with dementia and thereby make the disabilities associated with the development of dementia significantly more pronounced. These are depression, underactive thyroid gland (hypothyroidism), and visual and/or hearing impairments.

The diagnostic process leads to a formulation that brings together information from the various assessments and investigations and finally determines the likely cause of the observed clinical changes and sets them in the context of the individual. This is then the basis for developing an individualized care plan given the diagnosis and knowledge of the individual and his surroundings.

Incorporated in the CAMDEX-DS pack, are CAMDEX, DSM-IV, and ICD-10 criteria for dementia. Each set of criteria takes the form of a systematic checklist (as illustrated in Fig. 7.2). This is included as an aid to summarizing the information gained using the assessment schedule, as it relates directly to each criterion. The numbers of the relevant questions from the informant interview associated with each criterion are presented, and the amount of decline (slight or great) can be recorded. A judgment can then be made as to whether each criterion is met, and a diagnosis

	EVERYDAY SKILLS
A	Progressive failure in performance of the common activities of every day life, not due to impairment in health or physical handicap. General deterioration of mental processes manifest as impairment or loss of: • Skills necessary for usual activities at work, college, or day center • Ability to use household utensils and equipment

Area of Decline	Question		Slight Decline	Great Decline
Usual Daytime Activities	33	Usual daytime activities at work, college, or day center	↓ ☐	↓ ☐
	34	Special skill or hobby	↓ ☐	↓ ☐
Use of household Utensils / Equipment	36	Making a cup of tea	↓ ☐	↓ ☐
	37	Housework, e.g., dusting, dishwashing	↓ ☐	↓ ☐
	38	Preparing simple meals/snacks	↓ ☐	↓ ☐

40	Duration of changes greater than 6 months	Yes ☐

137–156	Changes due to ill health or physical handicap	No ☐

Criterion A Met	Yes ☐	No ☐

Fig. 7.2 Example diagnostic criterion

made on the basis of this information, in conjunction with information from physical and mental state examinations, cognitive assessments and other investigations. As stressed above, the aim of the CAMDEX-DS is not to provide a substitute for good clinical practice by rather to provide a framework to support the diagnostic process.

Guidance for Postdiagnosis Intervention

In recognition of the fact that the diagnosis of dementia marks the beginning rather than the end of a program of ongoing health and social care support, the CAMDEX-DS pack also includes a section providing guidance on postdiagnosis intervention. Dementia diagnosis is the starting point for the development of a detailed and integrated plan to meet the continually changing needs of the person with dementia and his or her family. The first part of this section provides a summary

Table 7.1 Summary of Guiding Principles for Postdiagnosis Intervention

1. Keep the person with dementia at the center of care planning
- Look at the person not the diagnosis and individualize care based on specific needs
2. Ensure all relevant people and agencies are working in partnership
- Family, advocates, GP, care manager, staff, professionals from community team
3. Forward thinking: prepare by being informed and anticipating change
- Consider where the person lives, daytime activities, training of care staff
4. Effective interventions, tailored to the individual
- Consider peer, family, and staff support, effective communication, memory books, interpreting challenging behaviors, environmental alterations, medication
5. Review and revise the person's needs and support strategies

of the key points that should be considered when planning support (outlined briefly in Table 7.1), while the second part consists of an example of an environmental checklist for residential homes, to help rate the suitability of the home for people with ID that develop dementia.

Review of Research Studies Using the CAMDEX-DS

The main application of CAMDEX-DS so far, has been its use in population-based research into dementia in people with DS. Diagnoses based on the informant interview that forms a major part of the CAMDEX-DS, have provided the basis for published estimates of the prevalence and incidence of dementia within this population. The informant interview and cognitive assessment (CAMCOG) have also been used longitudinally to chart the course of dementia in individuals who have been affected, providing valuable information regarding the sequence and timescale of decline in distinct areas of cognition, behavior, and functional ability.

Prevalence rates have been reported in the range of a few percent in those aged 30–39 years, between 10% and 25% in the 40–49 age group, between 20% and 50% in the 50–59 age group and between 30% and 75% in those over 60.[31–34] Variations in these rates can be explained in terms of differences in diagnostic criteria and selection bias in the subject groups studied. In an attempt to overcome these problems, Holland and colleagues[32] carried out an unbiased population-based study of individuals with DS using a slightly modified version of the CAMDEX informant interview to diagnose dementia using standard criteria (including ICD-10, DSM-IV, and CAMDEX criteria for DAT) and provisional criteria for frontal-type dementia (FTD).[35] Adults with DS over the age of 30 on July 1, 1994, within the catchment area (population 280,000), were identified through examination of health authority records, contact with community learning disability teams, contact with local private and voluntary services and direct contact with residential services for people with ID. Seventy-seven individuals met the inclusion criteria for the study and, of these, 75 agreed to take part.

Age-specific prevalence rates of dementia were found to vary according to the diagnostic criteria used, with more cases meeting CAMDEX compared to ICD-10[3] and DSM-IV[12] criteria. Using CAMDEX criteria for DAT, prevalence rates were found to increase from 3.4% in the 30–39 age group to 10.3% in 40–49 age group and to 40% in the 50–59 age group. These rates are similar to those observed in the general elderly population but shifted forward by 30–40 years. However, in addition to those participants who met criteria for DAT, a number of participants met provisional criteria for FTD, showing changes in personality or behavior in the absence of decline in memory. While age-specific prevalence rates for DAT were found to be higher in participants over 45 years of age, prevalence rates for FTD were higher in the younger age group (<45 years), a finding that was taken to suggest that the presentation of AD in people with DS may differ from that in the general population.

In a follow-up study, Holland and colleagues[36] used the modified CAMDEX informant interview to determine the extent and nature of changes in memory, personality, general mental functioning, and daily living skills over an 18-month period. At the first assessment, carers of 35 (71%) of the 49 participants for whom changes had been reported, stated that the first change they had noticed was in personality or behavior rather than in memory or other areas of functioning. At the second assessment, estimated incidence rates for a clinical presentation resembling FTD (characterized by personality/behavior changes) were shown to be high and greatest in the youngest age group, while incidence of DAT occurred predominately in the older group. On the basis of these findings, the authors hypothesized that functions served by the frontal lobes are the first to be compromised with the progressive development of Alzheimer-like neuropathology in people with DS, perhaps as a result of the known underdevelopment of this brain region in people with DS.[37] It was suggested that the lower reserve capacity of the frontal lobes in this population, may increase the vulnerability of frontal lobe functions to the effects of AD neuropathology resulting in a clinical presentation resembling that of FTD occurring prior to the development of the full features of AD. It is important to note that it is not suggested that individuals with DS develop FTD (which, in the general population, is associated with neuropathology that differs from that associated with AD) but that AD-like neuropathology results in a presentation similar to FTD in the early stages of AD in this population.

A further follow-up of the same population sample approximately 5 years later[38] has provided further support for this hypothesis. Dementia status was reassessed using the CAMDEX informant interview and documentation of progression in clinical presentation suggested that the clinical course of dementia begins with early changes in personality or behavior and is followed by an increase in characteristics associated with frontal lobe dysfunction, prior to the development of the full features of DAT. Participants who met criteria for FTD (with five or more reported changes in personality/behavior) were found to be at a significantly increased risk (1.5 times) of progressing to a diagnosis of DAT over the following 5 years compared to those who did not meet FTD criteria. What is more, participants whose personality and behavior changes were insufficient for a diagnosis of FTD (i.e., for whom 1–4 changes were reported) were found to be at a significantly increased risk (1.5 times) of progressing to a more severe diagnosis (e.g., FTD or DAT) over this period than those without such changes. This suggests that even limited evidence of change in personality or behavior is sufficient to increase the risk of dementia 5 years later.

In addition to examining clinical progression by way of informant reports, the CAMCOG cognitive assessment was completed at baseline and follow-up assessments, to provide a measure of decline in global cognitive function. Two additional measures were derived from the CAMCOG to examine specifically the sequence of decline in frontal lobe-associated EF and memory. The EF measure combined scores for the abstract thinking and attention/calculation subscales and scores for the verbal fluency item and the clock drawing item, which has been found to have a strong EF component.[39] The memory measure combined scores for the memory and orientation subscales. Degree of decline on these measures over the 5 years prior to diagnosis was compared across groups based on diagnosis and age. The sample was divided into five groups as follows: those who met CAMDEX criteria for DAT, those who met criteria for FTD, those who showed personality/behavior changes insufficient to meet FTD criteria, those with no reported changes who were younger than 50 years, and those with no personality/behavior changes who were older than 50 years.

Participants who met FTD criteria and those with 1–4 personality changes had shown a degree of decline on the CAMCOG that was intermediate between that of those with no reported changes and those with AD, and had shown a specific decline in EF with no significant decline on the memory measure. The DAT group, however, had shown a significant decline in both EF and memory over the preceding 5 years, but had show a significantly greater degree of decline in memory than in EF. These findings provide further support for the hypothesis that features similar to those associated with FTD are a precursor to the more marked cognitive deterioration associated with clinically diagnosed DAT. Interestingly, the group of older participants with no informant-reported changes decline to a greater degree than younger participants, but had shown a more generalized pattern of deterioration than individuals with informant-reported changes, with no significant difference in the degree of decline in EF and memory. This suggests that while age is likely to have an effect on cognitive function, such age-related changes appear to be distinguishable from preclinical AD.

The use of the modified CAMDEX in this longitudinal study has enabled the direct comparison of the clinical course of dementia in DS with that of dementia in the general population. This exploration of the differences and similarities that exist between the presentation of DAT in these two populations may serve to inform strategies for supporting individuals with DS who develop dementia and help to identify individuals at an early stage in the development of AD. This second benefit is likely to become increasingly important as new treatments become available that may halt or slow the progression of AD pathology.

In addition to the work carried out by Holland and colleagues, a number of other studies have also used the CAMDEX informant interview as a means of diagnosing dementia in this group. In a paper on the development of the Adaptive Behavior

Dementia Questionnaire (ABDQ),[40] a brief 15-item questionnaire tool for screening for dementia in DS, Prasher and colleagues report that the CAMDEX informant interview was used to aid the diagnosis of DAT according to ICD-10 criteria. This diagnosis served as the standard against which the validity of the ABDQ was established. Similarly, the usefulness of MRI as an aid to diagnosing DAT in people with DS was assessed by comparing MRI findings between individuals with and without clinically diagnosis of DAT (made using the CAMDEX informant interview) leading to the conclusion that the role of MRI was limited.[41] This method of diagnosis has also been used in a study investigating biological risk factors for dementia in DS. Rubenstein and colleagues[42] reported that apo-E genotypes are associated with similar risk effects in DS as they are in the general population, with apo-E4 allele carriers at increased risk of developing dementia (diagnosed on the basis of the CAMDEX informant interview) and apolipoprotein-E2 allele carriers at decreased risk.

In other studies, the CAMCOG assessment has been used as a measure of cognitive functioning in adults with ID. Beacher and colleagues[43] measured the association between concentration of myoinositol in the hippocampus and performance on the CAMCOG in older adults with DS and controls. The serum sodium/myoinositol cotransporter gene is located on chromosome 21, and myoinositol affects neuronal survival and function. In this study adults with DS were found to have significantly increased concentration of myoinositol compared to controls, and concentration of myoinositol was negatively correlated with cognitive performance. Prasher et al. (2005) suggest that further studies are required to relate myoinositol concentration to risk for AD in people with DS. Hassiotis and colleagues[44] describe the setting up of a memory clinic for older people with IBs, in which the CAMCOG is one of the instruments used to monitor cognitive function and decline over time.

Pros and Cons of the CAMDEX-DS

The major benefits of using the CAMDEX-DS to assess and diagnose dementia in people with DS are that (1) it enables the collection of information that maps directly onto standard diagnostic criteria for dementia; (2) it provides a structure for the collection of information regarding other potentially reversible disorders (e.g., depression), enabling a differential diagnosis to be made; (3) in relying on a formalized process for clinical diagnosis rather than a cutoff score, it enables the identification of individuals who may be suspected to be in the early or preclinical stages of dementia and who require close monitoring for further changes; and (4) it goes beyond diagnosis to provide guidance on intervention and support strategies for people with DS who are diagnosed with dementia.

However, the CAMDEX-DS is not a substitute for good clinical practice and does not eliminate the need for a full clinical assessment, with particular focus on those areas in which concern is highlighted through the use of the schedule. Clinical judgment remains the most important part of the diagnostic procedure. Furthermore, the schedule has been designed to provide a framework for a comprehensive dementia assessment and is therefore necessarily more time-consuming to administer than brief screening questionnaires.

While the CAMCOG direct cognitive assessment provides a quantitative score, which can be tracked longitudinally as an objective measure of decline, the diagnosis of dementia, based on the schedule as a whole, is a qualitative judgment so "degree of dementia" cannot be tracked in a quantitative manner as is the case for "scores" on dementia screening questionnaires. However progression in clinical presentation can be can be observed and reported on the basis of qualitative shifts over time.

Clinical Experience

Our experience in using this interview has been that carers and relatives of people with DS, who have known them for sometime are generally very perceptive to the subtle changes that occur in the person they care for abilities and behavior and, when prompted are able to provide specific examples of the kinds of changes that have occurred. In Appendix 6, three case studies are presented that show examples of changes in behavior reported by carers, obtained using the CAMDEX-DS informant interview.

Also presented, in Table 7.2, is a summary of how these reported changes map onto CAMDEX-DS criteria for DAT, illustrating the degree to which moving from

Table 7.2 Summary of Findings for Cases Mapped on CAMDEX-DS Criteria for DAT

CAMDEX-DS criteria for dementia of Alzheimer's type (DAT)	Case 1	Case 2	Case 3
Progressive failure of the common activities of everyday life	□	?	?
Decline in memory sufficient to impair functioning in daily life	□		?
Progressive impairment in cognitive functions other than memory	□	□	□
OR			
Deterioration of personality or general behavior	□	□	□
Clouding of consciousness/delirium not present most of the time	□	□	□
Gradual onset	□	□	□
Deterioration not accounted for by other disorders	□	? Hearing, depression	? Eyesight, depression, antiepileptic medication
Diagnosis	DAT	Does not meet DAT criteria—possible preclinical features	Possible DAT

specific examples of change to a diagnosis requires the use of clinical judgment, supported by the framework provided.

What these case studies illustrate is that the information gained from the inform-ant interview, may not in itself be sufficient to reach a diagnosis but may highlight areas of concern that need to be investigated before a diagnosis of dementia can be made or ruled out. In the case of Michael (Case 2) for example, the informant inter-view indicated that he suffered from a hearing impairment that was corrected by the use of a hearing aid. Such a finding should prompt an investigation as to whether the hearing aid is functioning properly or whether any reported changes could be due to hearing difficulties. The observation that he is now much more prone to cry-ing than he used to be, in conjunction with the fact that he is currently on antide-pressant medication should prompt a review of this medication and a full investigation into the presence of other features suggestive of depression.

In the case of Mary, who has a severe ID, the range of her abilities was so limited prior to any signs of dementia that it is difficult to establish whether deterioration has occurred. However, when prompted the carer was able to come up with specific examples of change, such as the fact that she has stopped singing songs (previously her favorite activity). Clinical judgment is required in order to conclude whether such changes are sufficient for diagnostic criteria to be met. Again, potential explanatory factors such as antiepileptic medication, features of depression and poor eyesight as a result of cataracts are highlighted as requiring further investigation.

Summary

With the changing age structure of populations, dementia and other illnesses related to old age are now the focus of very considerable research and policy attention in general. Given that people with DS have this high risk of DAT at a relatively young age their needs and the effectiveness of any new treatments for DAT must be con-sidered in this population. Reliable diagnosis and the ability to track decline is central to both treatment development and treatment trials and is also important in informing social care policy and support strategies. We believe that the following research and clinical issues require particular attention: (1) the identification of other individual or environmental risk or protective factors that modify the age of onset and course of dementia in people with DAT; (2) ethically and clinically sound trials in people with DS of treatments, as they are developed, aimed at the preven-tion or the amelioration of DAT; (3) the education and training of paid and family carers about the relationship between DS and DAT, how it presents, and what sup-port strategies are known to help maintain the quality of life of people with DS and dementia; and (4) the ultimate goal is establishing the underlying mechanism that accounts for the high risk of DAT in people with DS, and specifically whether overexpression of the amyloid precursor protein gene (located on chromosome 21) is the main etiological factor. Only then will new treatments be developed that are tailored specifically to people with DS. Each of these objectives, to varying degrees, requires the involvement of people with DS and their carers and the ability to detect with a high degree of certainty whether dementia is developing or has developed. Research therefore requires instruments such as the CAMDEX-DS and strong partnerships between people with DS, their families and paid carers, clinicians, and basic scientists.

References

1. Aylward E, Burt D, Thorpe L et al. (1997) Diagnosis of dementia in individuals with intellectual disability: Report of the task force for development of criteria for diagnosis of dementia in individuals with mental retardation. J Intellect Disabil Res 41: 152–164.
2. American Psychiatric Association (1994) Diagnostic and Statistical Manual of mental disorder. Washington DC: American Psychiatric Association.
3. World Health Organisation (1992) ICD-10 International Statistical Classification of Diseases and Related Health Problems, 10th edn. Geneva: WHO.
4. Roth M, Huppert FA, Mountjoy CQ et al. (1998) CAMDEX-R: The Cambridge Examination for Mental Disorders of the Elderly (Revised). Cambridge: Cambridge University Press.
5. Roth M, Tym E, Mountjoy C et al. (1986) CAMDEX—A standardised instrument for the diagnosis of mental disorder in the elderly with special reference to the early detection of dementia. Br J Psychiatry 149: 698–709.
6. Roth M, Huppert F, Tym E et al. (1988) CAMDEX: The Cambridge Examination for Mental Disorder of the Elderly. Cambridge: Cambridge University Press.
7. Neri M, Roth M, Vreese LPD et al. (1998) The Validity of Informant Reports in Assessing the Severity of Dementia: Evidence from the CAMDEX Interview. Dement Geriatr Cogn Dis 9: 56–62.
8. Huppert FA, Brayne C, Gill C et al. (1995) CAMCOG—A concise neuropsychological test to assist dementia diagnosis: Socio-demographic determinants in an elderly population sample. Br J Clin Psychol 34: 529–541.
9. Huppert FA, Jorm AF, Brayne C et al. (1996) Psychometric properties of the CAMCOG and its efficacy in the diagnosis of dementia. Aging Neuropsychol Cogn 3: 201–214.
10. Williams JG, Huppert FA, Matthews FE et al. (2003) Performance and normative values of a concise neuropsychological test (CAMCOG) in an elderly population sample. Int J Geriatr Psychiatry 18: 631–644.
11. Heinik J (1998) Effects of trihexyphenidyl on MMSE and CAMCOG scores of medicated elderly patients with schizophrenia. Int Psychogeriatr 10: 103–108.
12. Jobst K, Smith A, Szatmari M et al. (1992) Detection in life of confirmed Alzheimer's disease using a simple measurement of medial temporal lobe atrophy by computed tomography. Lancet 340: 1179–1183.
13. Clarke MCJ and Anderson J (1991) The prevalence of dementia in a total population: A comparison of two screening instruments. Aging 20: 396–403.
14. Cullum S, Huppert FA, McGee M et al. (2000) Decline across different domains of cognitive function in normal ageing: Results of a longitudinal population-based study using CAMCOG. Int J Geriatr Psychiatry 15: 853–862.
15. O'Connor D, Pollitt P, Hyde J et al. (1989) The prevalence of dementia as measured by the Cambridge Mental Disorders of the Elderly Examination. Acta Psychol Scand 79: 190–198.
16. Schmand B, Walstra G, Lindeboom J et al. (2000) Early detection of Alzheimer's disease using the Cambridge Cognitive Examination (CAMCOG). Psychol Med 30: 619–627.
17. Heinik J, Solomesh I, and Berkman P (2004) Correlation between the CAMCOG, the MMSE, and three clock drawing tests in a specialized outpatient psychogeriatric service. Arch Gerontol Geriatr 38: 77–84.

18. Nielsen H, Lolk A, Andersen K et al. (1999) Characteristics of elderly who develop Alzheimer's disease during the next two years—A neuropsychological study using CAMCOG: The Odense Study. Int J Geriatr Psychiatry 14: 957–963.
19. Forstl H, Burns A, Jacoby R et al. (1991) Neuroanatomical correlates of clinical misidentification and misperception in senile dementia of the Alzheimer type. J Clin Psychopharmacol 52: 268–271.
20. Gertz H, Xuereb J, Huppert F et al. (1996) The relationship between clinical dementia and neuropathological staging (BRAAK) in a very elderly community sample. Eur Arch Psychiatry Clin Neurosci 246: 132–136.
21. Cabranes J, De Juan R, Encinas M et al. (2004) Relevance of functional neuroimaging in the progression of mild cognitive impairment. Neurol Res 26: 496–501.
22. Hunter R, McLuskie R, Wyper P et al. (1989) The patterns of function-related cerebral blood flow investigated by single photon emission tomography with 99 m Tc-HMPAO in patients with presenile Alzheimer's Disease and Korsakoff's psychosis. Psychol Med 19: 847–855.
23. Lawton MP and Brody EM. (1969). Assessment of older people: Self-maintaining and instrumental activities of daily living. Gerontologist. 9: 179–186.
24. Saxton J, McGonigle KL, Swihart AA et al. (1993) The Severe Impairment Battery. Bury St. Edmunds: Thames Valley Test Company.
25. Witts P and Elders S (1998) The 'severe impairment battery': Assessing cognitive ability in adults with Down syndrome. Br J Clin Psychol 37: 213–216.
26. Ball SL, Holland AJ, Huppert FA et al. (2004) The modified CAMDEX informant interview is a valid and reliable tool for use in the diagnosis of dementia in adults with Down's syndrome. J Intellect Disabil Res 48: 611–620.
27. Deb S and Braganza J (1999) Comparison of rating scales for the diagnosis of dementia in adults with Down's syndrome. J Intellect Disabil Res 43: 400–407.
28. Landis JR and Koch GG (1977) The measurement of observer agreement for categorical data. Biometrics 33: 159–174.
29. Hon J, Huppert FA, Holland AJ et al. (1999) Neuropsychological assessment of older adults with Down's syndrome: An epidemiological study using the Cambridge Cognitive Examination (CAMCOG). Br J Clin Psychol 38: 155–165.
30. Folstein M, Folstein S, and McHugh P (1975) Mini-Mental State. A practical method for grading the cognitive state of patients for the clinician. J Psychol Res 12: 189–198.
31. Hewitt KE, Carter G, and Jancar J (1985) Ageing in Down's syndrome. Br J Psychiatry 147: 58–62.
32. Holland AJ, Hon J, Huppert FA et al. (1998) Population-based study of the prevalence and presentation of dementia in adults with Down's syndrome. Br J Psychiatry 172: 493–498.
33. Lai F and Williams RS (1989) A prospective study of Alzheimer disease in Down syndrome. Arch Neurol 46: 849–853.
34. Wisniewski KE, Wisniewski HM, and Wen GY (1985) Occurrence of neuropathological changes and dementia of Alzheimer's disease in Down's syndrome. Ann Neurol 17: 278–282.
35. Gregory CA and Hodges JR (1993) Dementia of frontal type and the focal lobar atrophies. Int Rev Psychiatry 5: 397–406.
36. Holland AJ, Hon J, Huppert FA et al. (2000) Incidence and course of dementia in people with Down's syndrome: Findings from a population-based study. J Intellect Disabil Res 44: 138–146.
37. Crome L and Stern L (1972) Pathology of Mental Retardation. Baltimore, MD: Williams and Wilkins.
38. Ball SL, Holland AJ, Hon J et al. (2006) Personality and behaviour changes mark the early stages of Alzheimer's disease in adults with Down's syndrome: Findings from a prospective population-based study. Int J Geriatr Psychiatry 21: 661–673.
39. Royall DR, Cordes JA, and Polk M (1998) CLOX: An executive clock drawing task. J Neurol, Neurosurg Psychiatry 64: 588–594.

40. Prasher VP, Farooq A, and Holder R (2004) The Adaptive Behaviour Dementia Questionnaire (ABDQ): Screening questionnaire for dementia in Alzheimer's disease in adults with Down syndrome. Res Dev Disabil 25: 385–397.
41. Prasher VP, Barber PC, West R et al. (1996) The role of magnetic resonance imaging in the diagnosis of Alzheimer disease in adults with Down syndrome. Arch Neurol 53: 1310–1313.
42. Rubinsztein DC, Hon J, Stevens F et al. (1999) Apo E genotypes and risk of dementia in Down Syndrome. Am J Med Genet B Neuropsychiatr Genet 88: 344–347.
43. Beacher F, Simmons A, Daly E et al. (2005) Hippocampal myo-inositol and cognitive ability in adults with Down syndrome: An in vivo proton magnetic resonance spectroscopy study. Arch Gen Psychiatry 62: 1360–1365.
44. Hassiotis A, Strydom A, Allen K et al. (2003) A memory clinic for older people with intellectual disabilities. Aging Ment Health 7: 418–423.

Chapter 8
The Test for Severe Impairment

N.M. Mulryan, J.F. Tyrrell, M. Cosgrove, E.M. Reilly, P. McCallion, and M. McCarron

Introduction

Langdon Down is reputed to have given the first comprehensive description of the eponymous syndrome in 1867.[1] Shortly after Down's paper, Fraser and Mitchell reported on a number of cases of "Kalmuc Idiocy" in which they refer to a "precipitated senility" seen in some of their subjects.[2] Due to the high mortality rates of those with Down syndrome (DS), disorders associated with advancing years were rarely seen in this era. Age-related health conditions have only become a particular issue in persons with intellectual disability (ID) and DS in recent decades, as they survive into the age of risk for developing dementia. Studying this subject has resulted in a greater understanding of the aging process in ID and in particular DS.[3–5]

Older persons with DS are uniquely at risk of developing Alzheimer's disease (AD) and account for about one-third of all people with ID who have dementia. It is projected that over the next 20 years, the biggest proportional increase in numbers of people with ID will be in the age group of over 55 years.[6] It is generally agreed that the prevalence of dementia in persons with DS exceeds that of the generic population and is estimated at 15% to 45% of persons with DS over 40 years of age.[7] An Irish study involving 285 subjects with DS, reported an age-specific prevalence of dementia at 5.7% in persons aged 40–49 years, 30.4% in persons aged 50–59 years, 41.7% in persons aged 60–69 years, and 50% in persons 70 years or older.[8] These reported rates are considerably higher than the rates reported in the general population aged 65 years and over.[9–11] The dementia prevalence in adults with ID other than DS has been reported to be 15.6% in persons aged 65–74 years, 23.5% in persons aged 75–84 years, and 70% in persons aged 85–94 years.[12] However, others report prevalence rates similar to the general population.[13]

The accurate and early diagnosis of dementia is important as it gives an opportunity to inform the individual and their carers of prognosis and treatment options. The advent of pharmacological interventions is a welcome development but their use requires knowledge of the disease stage and potential course of decline. Longitudinal assessment is advisable to facilitate the tracking of these changes and the impact of interventions.[14,15] Measurement of this decline has proved problematic, as

V.P. Prasher (ed.), *Neuropsychological Assessments of Dementia in Down Syndrome and Intellectual Disabilities*,
DOI: 10.1007/978-1-84800-249-4_8, © Springer Science+Business Media, LLC 2009

traditional tools such as the Mini-Mental State Examination (MMSE)[16] appear insensitive to tracking changes in the later stages of disease, particularly in those with ID.[17] Cognitive function may vary considerably between individuals and obtaining baseline measurements from which to assess change may be particularly fraught using traditional tools. Persons with DS are prone to developing dementia in Alzheimer's disease (DAD) at a young age therefore obtaining valid, reliable data is vital to ensure early intervention if required.

Burt and Aylward reported the findings of a working group, established under the auspices of International Association for the Scientific Study of Intellectual Disability (IASSID) and the American Association on Mental Retardation (AAMR), which proposed a battery of tests to aid the diagnosis of dementia in individuals with ID.[14] They identified that differentiating between changes associated with normal aging from dementia-related changes posed a significant challenge to Examiners. Both informant-based scales that report on an individual's functioning and tests for direct assessment were included in the proposed battery. The importance of inform-ant information was stressed, as was the need for longitudinal assessment. In order to establish a healthy baseline, the authors recommended that all individuals with DS should be assessed for the presence of dementia before the age of 40 years and before the age of 50 years for those with other causes of ID. Periodical reassessment should then occur depending on the age and symptoms of the individual.

Despite continued efforts in the development and validation of both informant-based (carer-rated) and objective test instruments (client-rated), as yet there is no agreed consensus on the optimal battery of test instruments to be used in detecting and diagnosing dementia in persons with varying degrees of ID. At present, the diagnosis of dementia in persons with ID remains a process of recognizing change from the person's previous level of functioning and then assessing that decline using available tools.

Development of Test for Severe Impairment

The Test for Severe Impairment (TSI) (see Appendix 7) was developed to provide a test of cognitive function for people with severe cognitive impairment.[18] The authors originally designed the test for use in the general population to measure function at an advanced stage of decline. In addition to being a valid and reliable tool, the test was designed to be nonthreatening, appealing, easily administered, time efficient and uses small readily available objects. The TSI is a 24-item cognitive test that takes 10 min to administer. It tests a broad range of cognitive functions and was designed for use in people from the general population whose MMSE score is less than 10 out of 30. The level of difficulty of the TSI is such that most people with moderate and severe ID should be able to score on it unless they are at an advanced stage of demen-tia. Also, a wide range of skills is tested including: language, memory, conceptual ability, and spatial skills. In total, the test contains six subsections each containing four items: well-learnt motor performance (fine and gross), language comprehension, language production, immediate and delayed memory, general knowledge, and conceptualization. Each item is either scored correct or incorrect. Each subsection has four questions, giving a total maximum score of 24, but the test was not designed to generate discrete subscale scores. Only eight out of the TSI's 24 items require the subject to answer a question verbally. This may be of benefit when testing persons with DS as their verbal abilities tend to be relatively poorly developed.

Albert and Cohen's original study involved 40 residents of a chronic care facility with a variety of types of dementia.[18] The MMSE was administered and only subjects scoring in the severe range (<11) were included in the study. Construct validity, external reliability, internal consistency, and factor structure were all studied proving the TSI to be a reliable and valid instrument. The internal consistency (alpha coefficient = 0.91) was considerably higher than that for the MMSE in the severe range ($a = 0.56$). It was suggested therefore that the TSI could complement the MMSE and give reliable scores for persons where the MMSE is exhibiting floor effects.

Foldi and colleagues[19] reassessed the TSI and compared it to the Dementia Rating Scale (DRS).[20] The DRS was developed to measure more severe impairment than the MMSE, however it requires training and time to administer making it less practical for use in a long-stay facility. They investigated the TSI's purported benefits from the perspectives of validity, reliability, and range. When criterion validity was calculated using the TSI and DRS total scores, the resulting correlation supported it being considered a valid screening tool ($r = 0.88$). A strong correlation was particularly noted in the memory and conceptualization domains, but weaker, nonsignificant correlations were found for language comprehension and production items. Indeed, when compared to the DRS scores the only item not to reach a significant level of correlation was the TSI item on language comprehension. Test–retest reliability and internal consistency reliability calculations both yielded high reliability scores. Further analysis suggested the TSI to be a tool applicable across a wide range of ability, not just for those with severe impairment. An additional aspect of this study correlated the TSI total score with the Boston Naming Test (BNT)[21] in an attempt to determine how well the TSI captures changes in naming skills. The total TSI and BNT scores correlated and in particular the language production score of the TSI correlated highly with the BNT. The authors suggested that the TSI may be of particular use when there are time constraints, more severe language impairment or the Examiner is not formally trained in psychological testing.

Jacobs and colleagues utilized the TSI in a longitudinal study of those with dementia but without ID.[22] Scores on the TSI were compared to results from the MMSE and the modified MMSE (mMMSE).[23] The mMMSE was constructed to strengthen perceived weaknesses in the MMSE, namely in the language, attention, and construction subsections. The TSI and the MMSE were found to be highly correlated ($r = 0.83$). Of particular note was the greater range of scores on the TSI for those obtaining very low scores on the MMSE. The mMMSE also correlated well with the TSI ($r = 0.82$). Those scoring in the severely impaired range of the mMMSE also produced a wide range of scores on the TSI, further supporting the relative robustness of the TSI in avoiding floor effects.

A modified version of the TSI (mTSI) was administered with the MMSE to 130 elderly females with moderate- to end-stage dementia but without ID.[24] In the modified version a facilitating cue was offered if the first response was incorrect; however, the number and content of the items were unchanged from the original TSI. Two points were scored for an outright correct answer and one point was offered for a correct answer following the facilitating cue. No points were given if the answer was incorrect or not given. Therefore the maximum score for the mTSI was 48 points. The mTSI score was different from zero significantly more often than the MMSE. In addition, only 9.2% of TSI items required a facilitating cue to give a correct answer. A limitation noted for both the MMSE and the mTSI was that approximately one-third of subjects were not tested due to behavioral concerns or the severity of their dementia. Appollonio surmised that this was likely to be a general limitation of performance-based instruments. A further study compared the performance-based mTSI with the observer-based Bedford Alzheimer Nursing Severity Scale (BANS-S).[25,26] Neither test was optimal, the mTSI appearing more useful in moderate to severe dementia, whereas the BANS-S mean scores only worsened in the later stages of the disease.

Validity and Reliability

Reports on the ease of administration and the likelihood of finding a range of scores among people with severe impairment suggested that the TSI might be a useful tool in the investigation of dementia in those with ID.[27] In an initial use of the TSI in the DS population, Cosgrave and colleagues assessed its validity and reliability in 60 older persons with DS.[28] The Down Syndrome Mental Status Examination (DSMSE) was administered in conjunction with the TSI. The DSMSE tests recall of personal information, orientation to season and day of the week, short-term memory, language, visuospatial construction, and praxis.[29] Comparing the results of both tests administered by the same rater indicated the convergent validity of the TSI for all subjects as 0.94. Interrater reliability for the TSI was satisfactory at 0.97 and test–retest reliability over 2 days yielded a concurrence of 0.98. Internal consistency of the TSI measured using Cronbach's alpha was 0.89. It was further reported that the TSI was brief and easy to administer and yielded a range of scores across all groups tested with the exception of those with severe ID and dementia. However, when compared with the DSMSE, the TSI provided a greater range of scores in the severe ID group. This finding in particular suggested the TSI would have greater utility as a tool in longitudinal testing, as it appeared less susceptible to the floor effects found in other instruments. Of concern, however, was that well-learned motor performances appeared to be retained until the later stages of the disease leading to recommendations that it should be used in conjunction with an observer-based rating instrument such as the Early Signs of Dementia Checklist.[30,31]

Rates of change on TSI scores in those with DAD in the general population were previously noted to be greatest in the middle stages of the disease with an average annual rate of change of 3 to 4 points.[22] Cosgrave and colleagues found a similar rate of score change of 3.2 points per year on the TSI in a 5-year study following

80 individuals.[30] However, the change was not linear with more modest reductions in early and late stages of dementia. The earliest items of the TSI to be affected in those with moderate ID and dementia included stating the number of weeks in the year, delayed memory, name writing, and counting to 10. In those with severe ID many items were answered incorrectly at the time of diagnosis except for learned motor responses. With the progression of dementia the last TSI item to be lost was shaking hands with the Examiner.

Tyrrell and colleagues also reported on the use of the TSI in a cross-sectional study of 285 persons with DS; of these, 185 lived in an institutional setting and 100 in the community.[8] At baseline testing, 38 cases of dementia were diagnosed according to DSM IV criteria giving a prevalence of 13.3%. The data gathered were subjected to logistic regression analysis yielding a model where scores on the Daily Living Scale Questionnaire (DLSQ), age and presence of epilepsy yielded the best fitting model for predicting dementia.[32] Neither the TSI nor DSMSE scores appeared predictive of dementia when analyzed in this manner. At year 2 there were 266 persons in the study including 46 persons with dementia, of whom 14 were newly diagnosed. Delayed and short-term memory, comprehension, and expressive language all appeared significantly impaired between year 0 and year 2. The annual rate of change of scores on the TSI was 1.4 (SD = ±2.6) for the dementia group and –0.35 (SD = ±1.2) for the nondementia group representing a significant difference (p = 0.0001). These changes were modest when compared with reports from the general population. Cosgrave and colleagues' findings with persons with DS also included a higher annual rate of change than calculated by Tyrrell and colleagues.[8,30] Tyrrell and colleagues' findings may reflect that the baseline scores may have included those who already had severe dementia and that the 24-month follow-up period was too short; detection of changes may require a longer time frame to become manifest.

The cohort studied by Cosgrave and colleagues is also important because it initiated a larger, longitudinal, and cross-sectional study. The 10 years of data collected to date in this larger study is presented here focusing on the findings in relationship to the TSI.

Methods

At time of entry into the study there were 80 women with DS living within the programs of one large service providers. The mean age of subjects at commencement was 47.7 years (SD 8.4, range 35–71 years). Thirty-nine of the subjects were living in long-stay residential type units, 24 subjects were living in a community setting, and 17 were living in campus group homes.

The same experienced clinician periodically assessed each subject over a 10-year period for the presence of dementia. Upon identification of symptoms, a dementia-specific team including a psychiatrist, psychologist, and physician reached consensus on the diagnosis of dementia using ICD criteria. Comorbid conditions likely to mimic dementia and known to be more common in aging persons with DS were ruled out as recommended by Pary.[33]

Measures

The TSI and the DLSQ were administered to all subjects. The TSI and its properties have been already described. The DLSQ is a 28-item test of adaptive behavior developed by the National Institute of Aging.[32] It is a carer-rated instrument and it covers the personal activities of daily living, as opposed to the instrumental activities of daily living. Previous application of this scale by this research group have indicated satisfactory psychometric properties with high correlation coefficients (0.83 and 0.95) on test–retest and interrater reliabilities for 32 subjects with DS and DAD. Further testing of the DLSQ with 60 subjects indicated a high correlation of this instrument (0.94) with the scores obtained on the TSI.[28] Following collection all data were coded and entered onto SPSS version 14.

Calculation of Rate of Change on TSI and DLSQ

The method utilized to calculate the annual rate of change on the TSI and DLSQ has been reported in previous longitudinal studies of this population[30] and was applied consistently here. Annual changes in scores for the entire follow-up period for each person regardless of dementia status was calculated by dividing the change in score over this time by the numbers of years of follow-up. Not all the data collected for each subject were used in this approach; however, the "restricted two-point estimate"[34] was deemed statistically more preferable. The results could have been skewed by uneven contributions as the number of assessments and time points differed by person.

For people with a previous diagnosis of dementia, a baseline score was utilized and was defined as the score in the year prior to the diagnosis of dementia or their year 1 score if they entered the cohort with dementia. The annual rate of change was calculated for those without dementia over their entire follow-up period. The scores of subjects whose scores had already "floored" were excluded from the analysis beyond that point as no further change was possible and further inclusion of scores would depress the change score of interest.

Temporal Stability of TSI and DLSQ

Temporal stability of the TSI and DLSQ was assessed using a *t*-test comparison of scores at baseline and follow-up on the TSI and DLSQ in persons with and without dementia.

Correlation Between Cognitive and Functional Changes

In order to understand if change in memory and cognition occurred simultaneously with change in global day-to-day functioning, scores on the TSI and DLSQ were correlated.

Results

Prevalence of Dementia

At baseline year (1996), seven cases were diagnosed with dementia, according to modified ICD-10 criteria, giving a prevalence of 8.7%. Over the following 10-year period the prevalence of dementia increased dramatically, with a total of 62 people (78.5%) meeting the criteria for dementia by the 10th year. The age of those with dementia was significantly older than persons without dementia (52.8 ± 8.2 vs. 44.8 ± 4.9 years, $t = -3.808$, $p < 0.001$, 95% CI (-12.18, -3.81). There was no difference in age of onset of dementia in persons with moderate ID vs. persons with severe ID (54.6 ± 6.7 vs. 51.4 ± 10.6 years). The duration of dementia was 5.2 (± 2.4) years. Of the total original population by the 10th year, 32 subjects had died and 31 of those still alive had a diagnosis of dementia.

Rates of Change on the TSI and the DLSQ

The mean annual rate of change of scores on the TSI was 1.8 (SD = ± 2.6) for the dementia group and -0.60 (SD = ± 1.4) for the nondementia group. The corresponding mean annual rate of change of scores on the DLSQ was 1.3 (SD = ± 1.4) for the dementia group and 0.28 (SD = ± 0.6) for the nondementia group.

Temporal Stability of TSI and DLSQ

t-Test comparisons of baseline and follow-up scores between subjects with and without dementia were significant for both the TSI ($p = 0.001$) and the DLSQ ($p = 0.006$).

Correlation Between Cognitive and Functional Changes

Scores on the DLSQ and the TSI were highly correlated at baseline and at diagnosis; the scores also being highly correlated with each other (Table 8.1). Consistent

Table 8.1 Correlation Table ADL (DLSQ) and TSI, Baseline and at Time of Diagnosis

		ADL at Diagnosis	Baseline ADL	TSI at diagnosis	Baseline TSI
ADL at diagnosis	Pearson correlation	1	.734 (**)	.769 (**)	.693 (**)
	Sig. (two-tailed)		.000	.000	.000
	N	40	40	38	38
Baseline ADL	Pearson correlation	.734 (**)	1	.701 (**)	.821 (**)
	Sig. (two-tailed)	.000		.000	.000
	N	40	73	38	65
TSI at diagnosis	Pearson correlation	.769 (**)	.701 (**)	1	.885 (**)
	Sig. (two-tailed)	.000	.000		.000
	N	38	38	39	39
Baseline TSI	Pearson correlation	.693 (**)	.821 (**)	.885 (**)	1
	Sig. (two-tailed)	.000	.000	.000	
	N	38	65	39	69

**Correlation is significant at the 0.01 level (two-tailed).

with these findings, scores on both scales at baseline and at their final administration were higher and remained higher for those without dementia as compared to those with dementia (Fig. 8.1). The scores were more likely to decline over time for those with dementia.

Discussion

Traditionally the MMSE has been viewed as an effective screening instrument for the general population. This instrument has not proved useful for persons with ID because often they already attain low scores because of their lifelong intellectual impairment. In the general population, scores on the MMSE also exhibit floor effects in later dementia. In consideration of this the TSI has been recommended as a more sensitive tool to measure change.[18] Use in both a cross-sectional[8] and a 5-year follow-up study[30] have already suggested that the TSI is a useful instrument for persons with DS. The findings here further support use of the TSI as a reliable and valid dementia test in this population. Given its properties, the tool has been used by a number of authors as part of neuropsychological evaluations of both general and ID groups.[35-46]

The administration of the TSI takes 10 min yet it assesses six different cognitive domains and the equipment is easy to carry and readily available. The test is short, easy to use and the findings here support that it is applicable across the range of dementia and levels of learning disability. The need for intact speech is minimized in comparison to other performance-based assessment tools and its range of use enhances its utility in longitudinal studies. However, the authors are concerned to emphasize that ease of use does not reduce the need for training in using the TSI to ensure consistency in application and scoring. A limitation is that the TSI was found here and in other studies to demonstrate a ceiling effect in persons with upper moderate and mild ID, and

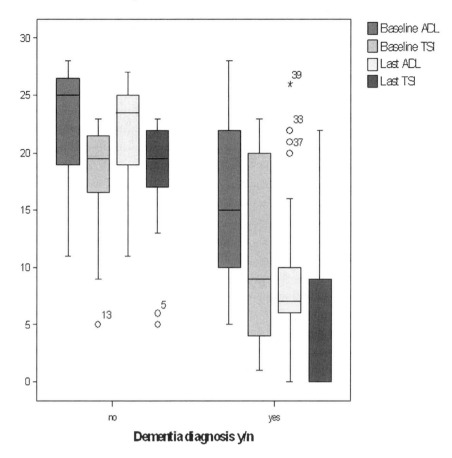

Fig. 8.1 Boxplot. Baseline ADL (DLSQ) TSI and latest TSI and ADL (DLSQ) scores by dementia

a floor effect in those with the most severe cognitive function. Yet this concern has been reported to be less prominent than in other instruments. Indeed, the TSI was found to produce a range of results in situations where subjects scored at or near zero in other tests. These are important findings; such sensitivity suggests for example that it may be feasible to use the TSI to monitor the effects of pharmacological interventions in dementia. As has been previously recommended,[14] the TSI should be augmented with an additional test of memory such as the Modified Fuld Object Memory Evaluation[47] and measures of functional ability.

Despite the reported strengths, the findings here are also consistent with other reports that a minority of subjects are unable to participate in testing due to severity of dementia or the presence of behavioral difficulties. Similar to floor effect concerns, this proportion however, appears to be less than with other tools and may be a general limitation of performance-based tools applied in end-stage dementia. The authors here also agree that sensory deficits such as color blindness or deafness may confound the administration of the TSI in a small proportion of subjects. A further limitation is that while the TSI provides gross evidence of decline, it gives no indication as to the potential cause. The content of the TSI may also benefit from slight alteration, as certain items such as stating the number of weeks in a year, appear universally difficult at baseline. In addition a measure of orientation would enhance the usefulness of the test without compromising its benefits.

Frequently with screening instruments clinical cutoff scores are established, sometimes to facilitate diagnosis and more often to support the need for additional assessment. Given the range of cognitive disability already present in persons with ID, creating such cutoff scores for the TSI would not be possible or useful. An alternative strategy has been to give greater attention to developing annual rate of change scores. In the general population the rate of change on TSI scores in those with mid-stage DAD have been reported as 3 to 4 points annually.[22] As was noted earlier, Cosgrave and colleagues reported a similar annual rate of change over 5 years for persons with DS.[30] However, Tyrrell and colleagues in a larger study found over 2 years a rate of change of approximately 1.4 per annum. The results reported in this chapter, following up on the Cosgrave and colleagues' sample at year 10, finds a rate more similar to Tyrrell and colleagues, i.e., 1.8 points per year for persons with dementia. More importantly the study confirms that for persons without dementia, there is no significant decline over time. Daily functioning scores for the group with dementia in this study also declined over time and for the group without dementia there is some decline but at a slower rate. The findings here do therefore indicate that declines over time in scores on the TSI are suggestive of dementia. Future investigation may elucidate whether annual assessments, prior to the onset of dementia, will further illustrate whether there is a decline in scores in the preclinical phase encouraging proactive screening. One factor that has not been accounted for in this study is the effect on the rate of decline of antidementia medications that have been introduced in recent years.

Summary

The longitudinal use of the TSI and the monitoring of rates of change appear to confirm its usefulness and to encourage the establishment of an early baseline for each individual to serve as a marker against which to compare later scores. Given these findings, the regular application of the TSI in clinical practice is recommended. However, measures of memory, adaptive behavior, and informant-based measures should be included to expand the clinical picture. When used in the advised manner the TSI appears to be a reliable and valid tool likely to aid in the diagnosis of dementia in those with ID.

Case Vignette

Ms. AB, a 44-year-old woman with DS, was referred for assessment to the Dementia Advisory Resource Center in 2002. At this time Ms. AB was living in a community residential setting with regular visits to her family home. She was artistically inclined, enjoyed socializing and worked in a craft center. A year prior to referral she was independent in self-care and was able to travel short distances alone by bus. Concerns raised by her carers regarding changes in her ability prompted further investigation.

At her initial assessment Ms. AB complained that she had occasionally missed her bus stop when traveling alone. She had also needed redirection at work as she returned to the incorrect table after lunch. In addition, she was annoyed that her carers supervised her dressing and she perceived this as an unnecessary intrusion. Apart from these issues she was content and denied any difficulties with sleep or appetite.

Collateral history from her family and carers indicated a progressive decline in cognitive and adaptive functioning in the previous year. She appeared disorientated at times, had difficulty in remembering recent events and required supervision when dressing. Her mood had remained stable and there was no evidence of biological symptoms of depression. Ms. AB was diagnosed with hypothyroidism in 1999 and was compliant with treatment. Premorbidly Ms. AB was independent in her daily activities. She enjoyed helping out with household chores and would travel independently to attend work. She socialized with her work colleagues at weekends when they would go to the movies or shops.

Following her initial interview, Ms. AB had a battery of blood tests to rule out possible underlying medical conditions that may present in a similar manner. No significant abnormalities were found. An electroencephalogram performed some time later was grossly normal, whereas a brain computerized tomography scan showed diffuse atrophy.

Ms. AB completed a battery of neuropsychological tests to assess her basic cognitive and functional skills. The results of these tests were compared to previous results obtained premorbidly in 2000. The results of these and subsequent tests are presented in Table 8.2

Ms. AB's clinical information was collated and presented to a clinical multidisciplinary group to discuss the diagnosis of dementia and to plan both pharmacological and psychosocial interventions.

Following diagnosis a choline-esterase inhibitor was commenced and a care plan devised to deal with her particular needs. A year after her diagnosis Ms. AB suffered a tonic-clonic seizure that required investigation in a general hospital. She often forgot the names of familiar staff and became increasingly frustrated with dressing and performing routine tasks. She became fixated with toilet rolls and

Table 8.2

Date	2000	2002	2003	2004	2005	2006	2007
DSMSE	20	18	10	5	1	0	0
TSI	21	20	13	8	5	1	0
DLSQ	20	11	7	2	1	0	0

DSMSE, Down Syndrome Mental State Examination; TSI, Test for Severe Impairment; DLSQ, Daily Living Skills Questionnaire.

appeared to be moody. The following year she was unable to recognize photos in an album and was experiencing difficultly in sequencing multistaged tasks. She was reported to be frequently tearful and anxious and her mood was becoming increasingly labile. Her mobility decreased, making outings problematic as she would lean on staff and tend to fall forward.

By 2005, Ms. AB was reported to be occasionally incontinent of urine, a problem compounded by her distress at bathing. She no longer recognized familiar faces and would hit out at people. Although still residing in a community house her level of dependence increased as her mobility and self-care decreased. Although free of tonic-clonic seizures for over a year she had episodes of myoclonus on wakening.

The following year Ms. AB was moved to a residential setting where her needs could be better addressed. She was dependent in all activities, was doubly incontinent and required 24-hour care. Mobilization by hoist was facilitated by her relative placidity. In view of the stage of dementia her family and carers discussed plans for her management in the end stage of her illness.

The 2007 assessment proved difficult, as Ms. AB was no longer able to cooperate with testing. Her physical health had shown a marked decline with a number of infections treated in the previous months. She was reported to be content and free of discomfort. It is unlikely than further formal assessments will be possible, however the dementia service will maintain its involvement in an advisory capacity in relation to day-to-day and end of life matters.

Regular involvement of a dementia service ensured that specialist advice was available to carers and family. In addition to providing practical guidance, the service guarantees regular assessment of cognitive and functional abilities. In Ms. AB's case a baseline assessment was performed prior to the identification of decline. This facilitated the diagnosis of dementia and allowed measurement of change from this point. All the instruments used demonstrated a falling off in scores over time. These measures reflected the clinical picture; however, both the DSMSE and DLSQ showed floor effects earlier than the TSI. The benefit of using a battery of tests is important as they assess a number of domains that deteriorate at differing rates. Further development of tools may allow assessment in the later stages of dementia enhancing the growth of knowledge of this disease.

References

1. Down JLH (1867) Observation on an ethnic classification of idiots. *J Ment Sci* 13: 121–3.
2. Fraser J and Mitchell A (1876) Kalmuc Idiocy: A report of case with autopsy. *With notes on sixty-two cases. J Ment Sci* 98: 168–79.
3. Burt DB, Primeaux-Hart S, Loveland KA et al. (2005) Aging in adults with intellectual disabilities. *Am J Ment Retard* 110: 268–84.
4. McCarron M, Gill M, McCallion P et al. (2005) Health co-morbidities in ageing persons with Down syndrome and Alzheimer's dementia. *J Intellect Disabil Res* 49: 560–6.
5. Holland AJ (2000) Ageing and learning disability. *Br J Psychiatry* 176: 26–31.
6. Barron S, Kelly C (2006) National Intellectual Disability Database Committee Annual Report. Dublin: Health Research Board.

7. Prasher VP and Krishnan VHR (1993) Age of onset and duration of dementia in people with Down syndrome: Integration of 98 reported cases in the literature. *Int J Geriatr Psychiatry* 8: 915–22.
8. Tyrrell J, Cosgrave M, McCarron M et al. (2001) Dementia in people with Down's syndrome. *Int J Geriatr Psychiatry* 16: 1168–74.
9. Hofman A, Rocca WA, Brayne C et al. (1991) The prevalence of dementia in Europe: a collaborative study of 1980–1990 findings. *EURODEM Prevalence Research Group. Int J Epidemiol* 20: 736–48.
10. Rocca WA, Hofman A, Brayne C et al. (1991) Frequency and distribution of Alzheimer's disease in Europe: a collaborative study of 1980–1990 prevalence findings. *The EURODEM-Prevalence Research Group. Ann Neurol* 30: 381–90.
11. Von Strauss E, Viitanen M, De Ronchi D et al. (1999) Aging and the occurrence of dementia: Findings from a population-based cohort with a large sample of nonagenarians. *Arch Neurol* 56: 587–92.
12. Cooper SA (1997) High prevalence of dementia among people with learning disabilities not attributable to Down's syndrome. *Psychol Med* 27: 609–16.
13. Janicki MP and Dalton AJ (2000) Prevalence of dementia and impact on intellectual disability services. *Ment Retard* 38: 276–88.
14. Burt DB and Aylward EH (2000) Test battery for the diagnosis of dementia in individuals with intellectual disability. *J Intellect Disabil Res* 44: 175–80.
15. Yesavage JA and Brooks III JO (1991) On the importance of longitudinal research in Alzheimer's disease. *J Am Geriatr Soc* 39: 942–4.
16. Folstein MF, Folstein SE, McHugh PR (1975) Mini-mental state. A practical method for grading the cognitive state of patients for the clinician. *J Psychol Res* 12: 189–98.
17. Deb S and Braganza J (1999) Comparison of rating scales for the diagnosis of dementia in adults with Down's syndrome. *J Intellect Disabil Res* 43: 400–7.
18. Albert M and Cohen C (1992) The Test for Severe Impairment: An instrument for the assessment of patients with severe cognitive dysfunction. *J Am Geriatr Soc* 40: 449–53.
19. Foldi NS, Majerovitz SD, Sheikh K et al. (1999) The Test for Severe Impairment: Validity with the Dementia Rating Scale and utility as a longitudinal measure. *Clin Neuropsychol* 13: 22–9.
20. Mattis S (1988) Dementia Rating Scale: Professional Manual. Odessa, FL: Psycho Assess Resources.
21. Mack W, Freed D, Williams BW et al. (1992) Boston Naming Test: Shortened version for use in Alzheimer's disease. *J Gerontol: Psychol Sci* 47: P154–8.
22. Jacobs DM, Albert SM, Sano M et al. (1999) Assessment of cognition in advanced AD: The test for severe impairment. *Neurology* 52: 1689–91.
23. Stern Y, Sano M, Paulson J et al. (1987) Modified Mini-mental State Examination: Validity and reliability. *Neurology* 37(S1): 179.
24. Appollonio I, Gori C, Riva GP et al. (2001) Cognitive assessment of severe dementia: The Test for Severe Impairment (TSI). *Arch Gerontol Geriatr* 7(Suppl): 25–31.
25. Appollonio I, Gori C, Riva G et al. (2005) Assessing early to late stage dementia: The TSI and BANS-S scales in the nursing home. *Int J Geriatr Psychol* 20: 1138–45.
26. Volicer L, Hurley AC, Lathi DC et al. (1994) Measurement of severity in advanced Alzheimer's disease. *J Gerontol* 49: M223–6.
27. Tyrrell JF, Cosgrave MP, McLaughlin M et al. (1996) Dementia in an Irish population of Down's syndrome people. *Ir J Psychol Med* 13: 51–4.
28. Cosgrave MP, McCarron M, Anderson M et al. (1998) Cognitive decline in Down syndrome: A validity/reliability study of the Test for Severe Impairment. *Am J Ment Retard* 103: 193–7.
29. Haxby JV (1989) Neuropsychological evaluation of adults with Down's syndrome: Patterns of selective impairment in non-demented old adults. *J Ment Defic Res* 33: 193–210.
30. Cosgrave MP (2000) Clinical and biological aspects of dementia in Down's syndrome. MD thesis, Shelf mark 5643, University of Dublin, Trinity College Dublin, Ireland.

31. Visser FE and Kuilman M (1990) Dementia symptoms in Down's syndrome in a residentially treated group of mentally handicapped. *Nederlands Tijdschrift voor Geneeskunde* 134: 1141–5.
32. National Institute of Aging, Laboratory of Neurosciences (1989) The Daily Living Skills Questionnaire. National Institute of Aging, US.
33. Pary R (1992) Differential diagnosis of functional decline in Down's syndrome. *The Habilitative Mental Healthcare Newsletter.* 11: 37–41.
34. Stern RG, Mohs RC, Bierer LM et al. (1992) Deterioration on the Blessed test in Alzheimer's disease: longitudinal data and their implication for clinical trials and identification of subtypes. *Psychol Res* 42: 101–10.
35. Bird TD, Nochlin D, Poorkaj P et al. (1999) A clinical pathological comparison of three families with frontotemporal dementia and identical mutations in the tau gene (P301L). *Brain* 122: 741–56.
36. Cosgrave MP, Tyrrell J, McCarron M et al. (1999) Determinants of aggression, and adaptive and maladaptive behaviour in older people with Down's syndrome with and without dementia. *J Intellect Disabil Res* 43: 393–9.
37. Silver MH, Newell K, Brady C et al. (2002) Distinguishing between neurodegenerative disease and disease-free aging: Correlating neuropsychological evaluations and neuropathological studies in centenarians. *Psychosom Med* 64: 493–501.
38. Breuer B, Martucci C, Wallenstein S et al. (2002) Relationship of endogenous levels of sex hormones to cognition and depression in frail, elderly women. *Am J Geriatr Psychiatry* 10: 311–20.
39. McCarron M, Gill M, Lawlor B et al. (2002) A pilot study of the reliability and validity of the Caregiver Activity Survey—Intellectual Disability (CAS-ID). *J Intellect Disabil Res* 46: 605–12.
40. Zigman WB, Schupf N, Devenny DA et al. (2004) Incidence and prevalence of dementia in elderly adults with mental retardation without Down syndrome. *Am J Ment Retard* 109: 126–41.
41. Silverman W, Schupf N, Zigman W et al. (2004) Dementia in adults with mental retardation: Assessment at a single point in time. *Am J Ment Retard* 109: 111–25.
42. Burt DB, Primeaux-Hart S, Loveland KA et al. (2005) Comparing dementia diagnostic methods used with people with intellectual disabilities. *J Policy Practice Intellect Disabil* 2: 94–115.
43. Burt DB, Primeaux-Hart S, Loveland KA et al. (2005) Aging in adults with intellectual disabilities. *Am J Ment Retard* 110: 268–84.
44. Cooper SA, Smiley E, Morrison J et al. (2007) Mental ill-health in adults with intellectual disabilities: Prevalence and associated factors. *Br J Psychiatry* 190: 27–35.
45. Pyo G, Kripakaran K, Curtis K et al. (2007) A preliminary study of memory tests recommended by the Working Group for individuals with moderate to severe intellectual disability. *J Intellect Disabil Res* 51: 377–86.
46. Cooper SA, Smiley E, Morrison J et al. (2007) An epidemiological investigation of affective disorders with a population-based cohort of 1023 adults with intellectual disabilities. *Psychol Med* 37: 873–82.
47. Seltzer GB (1997) Modified Fuld Object Memory Evaluation. Waisman Centre, University of Wisconsin, Madison, WI.

Chapter 9
The Cued Recall Test: Detection of Memory Impairment

D.A. Devenny and S.J. Krinsky-McHale

Introduction

Memory decline is a characteristic of normal aging as well as an early symptom of dementia in Alzheimer's disease (DAD) in both individuals from the general population and in individuals with intellectual disability (ID). The determination of decline in individuals with ID is difficult because they have a compromised memory system even when young and healthy. The Cued Recall Test, a list-learning task that presents test items in a controlled learning paradigm, has both concurrent and predictive validity and is promising as a research and as a clinical diagnostic measure for the identification of memory impairment in adults with ID.

The first issue we address is the identification of memory impairment associated with DAD in individuals with Down syndrome (DS). The diagnosis of DAD was made by community physicians independent of the findings of the Cued Recall Test. Both cross-sectional and longitudinal findings show that the Cued Recall Test can discriminate individuals with DAD from those without the diagnosis. The second issue is the identification of memory impairment in individuals with DS prior to a diagnosis of DAD. Longitudinal data indicated progressive declines in performance on the Cued Recall Test in some individuals, suggesting that they may be in a preclinical phase of the disease. Finally we examined the effectiveness of the Cued Recall Test in detecting changes associated with normal aging in adults with DS. Older adults were poorer on the free recall of test items, one of the component measures of this test.

Background

Memory impairment is a behavioral signature of DAD and is frequently the first sign of change in individuals from the general population.[1,2] Establishing an "impairment" in individuals with ID is difficult because performance on memory tasks is related to level-of-cognitive functioning which varies considerably among these individuals. Setting a level for "impairment," then, is problematic when

V.P. Prasher (ed.), *Neuropsychological Assessments of Dementia in Down Syndrome and Intellectual Disabilities*,
DOI: 10.1007/978-1-84800-249-4_9, © Springer Science+Business Media, LLC 2009

baseline memory ability is compromised. In spite of these problems in measure-ment, recent longitudinal studies have determined that, as in the general population, memory impairment is also one of the first signs of change associated with DAD in adults with (DS).[3-5]

Performance on memory tasks not only depends on memory ability but is influenced by other cognitive abilities, such as attention, processing capacity and efficient use of strategies,[6] abilities which show attenuation with normal aging and which may be selectively or globally impaired in individuals with ID at any age. In the general population, procedures that induce semantic processing (e.g., providing category cues for test items) have been shown to reduce the influence of these other cognitive abilities on memory in healthy older adults and thus reduce the overall effects of aging on memory tasks. These category cues are most efficient when they are provided both as a support for encoding and for retrieval.[7] In a typical para-digm of controlled learning, items on a memory task are introduced with a category cue and the same cue is provided when initial spontaneous retrieval of an item fails.[6,8,9] That is, the encoding of each task item is enhanced by focusing attention on a semantic association, and retrieval is enhanced by its close alignment with the context of encoding. While there have been several variations of this paradigm, the procedure, in general, has been found to be effective in identifying specific mem-ory impairment associated with Alzheimer's disease (AD) in older adults from the general population.[8-12]

For the past 10 years we have administered a memory test that employs a controlled learning paradigm[13] that was modeled on a procedure developed by Grober and Buschke.[14] This memory test is included in a neuropsychological test battery in a longitudinal study of aging among individuals with ID. In this study we are particularly interested in the course of aging among adults with DS as both premature aging and a high risk for AD are associated with this syndrome. The goals of the study are to examine changes in cognitive functioning associated with normal aging and to distinguish these changes from those associated with early-stage dementia. Since declines in memory are one of the primary and earliest signs of change in dementia, we focused our efforts on evaluating and developing tasks that could detect the earliest changes in memory and in identifying areas of cogni-tive ability that influence memory performance.

Identification of Memory Impairment in Adults with Dementia in the General Population

Memory measures found to be most sensitive to age-associated declines focus primarily on episodic memory. Episodic memory is related to the acquisition of information obtained in a specific time and place[15] and is dependent on the integ-rity of the hippocampus and its connections with the frontal lobe.[16] List-learning tasks are used to assess this type of memory; the items on the list, while within the vocabulary of the individual, are uniquely associated with the event of the specific testing situation. In the controlled learning paradigm the items to be recalled are presented with a category cue that is related to the test item. In the learning phase there is an opportunity to learn the test items over repeated trials. In the testing phase, for each trial, free recall is followed by cued recall in which the category cue is provided for each item that was not recalled spontaneously.

Initial studies of the cued recall procedure found that it discriminated between individuals with and without a diagnosis of DAD.[2,8,14] In a version with a maximum score of 48, a cutoff score of ≤44 identified all participants who had a diagnosis of dementia.[6] Because the presence of the category cue was so effective in facilitating retrieval in individuals who did not have dementia, Grober and Kawas[9] found a ceiling effect in using the Total Score (Free Recall + Cued Recall) in individuals who were in a preclinical phase of DAD. Follow-up testing 3 years later, however, showed a deficit for those participants with DAD relative to healthy elderly control participants.

In order to make the test more difficult and to eliminate the ceiling effect, Buschke and colleagues[8] modified the procedure in the cued recall task by increasing the number of items to 64 and providing four exemplars for each of the 16 categories. This modified version of the task provided good sensitivity and specificity in distinguishing individuals with mild DAD from healthy participants. The controlled learning procedure, then, facilitates encoding specificity in older, healthy adults but is not able to overcome the memory deficit associated with DAD.

Age-Associated Memory Impairment and Down Syndrome

In adults with DS, the effects of aging on the memory system are imposed on a cognitive organization that has an atypical developmental history.[17] Although the investigation of the memory system in relation to aging in adults with ID is relatively recent, initial findings show a pattern of performance that mirrors that seen in the general population. In longitudinal studies, older adults with DS showed small age-related declines in episodic memory[5,13,18–20] and recent cross-sectional studies have shown that older adults with DS are poorer than their younger peers on measures of visual short-term memory.[21–23] In contrast, auditory short-term memory span shows little or no decline either with normal aging[3,4,19] or with early-stage dementia in adults with DS.[3]

Diagnosis of Early-Stage Dementia in Adults with Down Syndrome

Declines in episodic memory are frequently the earliest symptom of change associated with DAD and are distinguished from declines associated with normal aging by the degree of impairment.[13,20] Identifying the early stages of dementia with neuropsychological tests is difficult because dementia has an insidious onset, there is heterogeneity of initial cognitive deficits, and many areas of early deficits are shared with normal aging and with dementia from other causes.[24] In adults with DS there is the additional difficulty of distinguishing changes in cognitive function associated with dementia from those related to precocious but normal aging, and from those attributable to lifelong cognitive impairments. Typically, baseline measures from which to assess change are unlikely to be available for most patients seen in diagnostic clinics. Because we employed a longitudinal study design, we were able to use individuals as their own controls and to look for the sequence and magnitude of decline on multiple measures of cognition and memory. One aim of our study, then, has been to develop tests that will be clinically useful when administered as a one-time measure to identify memory impairment.

Early Identification of Significant Memory Impairment in Adults with Down Syndrome

A second aim of our study has been to develop measures that will identify individuals with DS who have Mild Cognitive Impairment (MCI). In the general population, MCI refers to an acquired significant memory impairment, while skills of daily living and general cognition remain intact.[25,26] MCI is a relatively recent classification term and implies that the observed changes in memory are in excess of what would be expected with normal aging. In addition, studies have shown that deficits in higher cognitive abilities associated with language, judgment and problem solving may coexist with memory deficits.[27-29] Identifying MCI is of interest because for some individuals it represents the early preclinical period for DAD. Individuals from the general population who are identified as having MCI appear to be at higher risk for developing dementia than older adults without significant memory declines. When MCI was based on memory impairment, an estimated rate of annual conversion from MCI to DAD ranged from 6% to 25%[26,29,30]; however, in individuals when memory impairment was accompanied by declines in additional cognitive abilities the conversion rate increased to a range of 40% to 60%.[28,29,31]

The distinction between MCI and a "preclinical" stage of dementia is currently far from clear. "Preclinical" refers to the period of cognitive decline prior to when an individual meets the criteria for a diagnosis of dementia and is estimated to have a duration from 6 to10 years.[27,32] Although a cognitive profile of deficits may not easily distinguish prospectively between MCI and preclinical DAD, retrospectively it is possible to evaluate decline from the time of diagnosis of dementia and determine those individuals who were "preclinical." The sequence of cognitive decline associated with both MCI and preclinical DAD appears to have some regularity, with deficits in memory, and particularly delayed recall, occurring several years before diagnosis.[27,32] Intervention at this stage to prolong the period before the onset of dementia is a goal of many recent clinical trails.[25]

Identifying MCI in adults from the general population is based on a premise of being able to define a narrow expected range of "normal" memory functioning. A specified deviation from what is defined as "normal," then, constitutes memory impairment. In adults with DS this premise is untenable because of the variability in their initial baseline level-of-functioning. However, despite this variability, recent longitudinal studies have shown that our measures of memory that have been adapted for use with adults with DS are able to identify individuals with significant memory declines.[13,20]1

Measures of Episodic Memory in Adults with Down Syndrome

The first test of episodic memory we administered, the Selective Reminding Test (SRT), consisted of eight items from a single category (food or animals). On the first trial of this test, the items were presented auditorily and the participant was asked to recall them. On each of the subsequent five trials, the participant was reminded of only those items not recalled on the previous trial. We have administered this test at each 12- to 18-month assessment cycle for the past 19 years of our longitudinal study. We have found this to be a test with good reliability[18] and with the ability to detect age-associated decline in memory when administered longitudinally.[18,20] We were also able to specify significant decline in memory associated with early-stage dementia. We have established a criterion of a 20% decline from an individual's previous highest score for two consecutive years as indicating the amount of decline associated with early-stage dementia.[20] This criterion, however, relies on having at least one baseline score that is representative of the individual's memory ability on this test, administered at a time when the individual was healthy and free from dementia, and on having two subsequent evaluations conducted over a 2-year period.

Ten years ago we introduced the Cued Recall Test into our battery. This is also a list-learning task, but differs from the SRT in some critical elements. The Cued Recall Test has an increased number of items (12 test items), and each item is from a different semantic category. In addition, the Cued Recall Test facilitates the encoding of items into storage because there is an initial learning phase in which items are systematically presented in small units (four at a time), the test items are presented both auditorily and visually (picture format), and participants are re-presented with the category cue that was provided in the learning phase if they are unable to spontaneously retrieve an item. This category cue, if efficiently utilized

---

1In our longitudinal study only a small number of individuals with ID from unknown etiologies have received a diagnosis of DAD. These individuals showed the same pattern of memory decline as we have reported for individuals with DS and their scores on the Cued Recall Test were ≤23 at the time of their diagnosis. Because there were so few individuals in this group we can only suggest that the Cued Recall Test will be applicable to the identification of significant memory impairment in this group.

by the participant, constrains the internal search for a test item and may prompt recognition, a component of memory that is less vulnerable to declines associated with normal aging.

Procedure

We modeled the Cued Recall Test on a measure developed by Grober and Buschke that identifies memory problems in adults from the general population.[14,33] The stimuli are 12 black and white line drawings[34] with each item represen-ting a distinct semantic category. There are two versions of the test that are alternated across test cycles in our longitudinal study (see Devenny and collea-gues[13] for specific test items). In comparison with the original test for the general population, we chose items and categories appropriate for the vocabulary of individuals with mild and moderate ID, we reduced the number of items from 16 to 12, and we modified the training procedures. In our procedure, the partici-pant is presented with the category cue only once during the initial presentation of the items. If any subsequent learning trials are required only the specific name of the item is repeated. This procedure focuses on the learning of the specific names for each test item.

The testing procedure for the Cued Recall Test involves a learning phase and a testing phase. In the learning phase the goal is to achieve encoding specificity by providing the participant with the same category cues that will be used to prompt retrieval. Four pictures are presented at a time, one in each quadrant of an 8″ × 11″ card and the participant is asked to inspect the card and name the picture corres-ponding to the verbal category cue (e.g., "Which one is fruit?") (Fig. 9.1). After the participant has pointed to and named each of the four items, the card is removed and he is asked to immediately recall the four test items from memory. Presentation of the cards for the learning of the items ceases when all four items are correctly recalled, or after three trials of the presentation of each card.[2] After the learning phase the stimuli are removed from the view of the participant.

The testing phase immediately follows completion of the learning phase and consists of three trials of free and cued recall. Each trial begins by asking for free recall of all 12 test items in any order. The free recall portion of a trial ends when the individual either indicates that he/she does not remember any more items or the individual begins to repeat items already named. For each item not recalled during the free recall trial, the category cue is provided (e.g., "What was the animal?") and the individual is given the opportunity to respond. This acts as a focused reminder

---

[2]The number of items that are recalled on each trial is noted. Typically, the four items are learned by the third trial. If, however, by the third trial all the items are not recalled, the participant is shown the card one more time with the absent item(s) pointed out, but no further recall trials are given for that card.

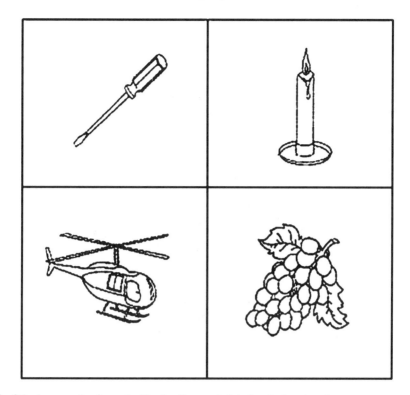

Fig. 9.1 An example of a card with stimuli presented during the learning phase

and in individuals without significant memory impairment the category cue is usually sufficient to prompt the recall of the specific item. If the individual does not retrieve the item with the cue, the participant is reminded of the missed item (e.g., "The animal was a rabbit."). Two scores are generated for each trial, a Free Recall Score and a Total Score (Free Recall Score + Cued Recall Score).

Participant Characteristics

Participants in our longitudinal study consisted of adults with DS and those with ID with unspecified etiologies. Inclusion criteria for the study are: (1) no suspicion by caregivers of declines in functioning; (2) no uncorrected serious sensory impairments; (3) absence of uncontrolled seizure disorder; (4) age ≥30 years; (5) IQ ≥ 30; (6) attendance at a community program, such as independent employment, workshop or day treatment program.

During the course of the study, three individuals developed chronic medical conditions that could contribute to a profile of cognitive decline (clinical depression, stroke, and transient ischemic attacks) and these individuals were eliminated

Table 9.1 Participant Characteristics of Etiology and Mean Age and IQ with Standard Deviations in Parentheses

Etiology	Status	N	Age	IQ
Unspecified ID	Healthy	61	59.2 (11.7)	58.4 (11.5)
	DAD	1	75.7	86
	MCI	2	58.2 (10.7)	58.5 (5.0)
Down syndrome (DS)	Healthy	61	48.2 (8.3)	54.2 (11.2)
	DAD	32	55.4 (5.4)	53.6 (11.2)
	MCI	14	52.6 (6.8)	48.5 (10.4)

from our analyses. Over the course of the study 32 individuals with DS have developed dementia. A diagnosis of DAD was provided by a physician once declines in memory, other cognitive abilities and activities of daily living were established and other causes of decline were ruled out. Among participants with ID from unspecified etiologies, one individual has received a diagnosis of DAD. In addition, we have some individuals who have substantial declines in memory ($N = 14$ with DS; $N = 2$ with unspecified etiologies) that suggest they may be in the preclinical period and we have identified them as having MCI (Table 9.1).

Participants were divided into those with DS and those with an ID that does not have a known etiology. A status of "healthy" indicates that no declines have been identified in cognitive/memory or adaptive functioning. DAD was diagnosed by a physician. A MCI indicates significant memory impairment without declines in adaptive functioning.

Psychometric Properties

Reliability of Different Versions of the Test

For the past 6 years we have alternated between two versions of the Cued Recall Test.[13] Our first assessment was to determine if the two versions were comparable. We examined the scores from 95 individuals (with DS and with unspecified ID) who have remained healthy over this period and for whom we had at least three sets of scores within the first three test cycles. A comparison of the two different test versions administered approximately 1.5 years apart showed a Pearson correlation coefficient of 0.564 for the Total Score ($p < .001$) and a coefficient of 0.469 for the Free Recall Score ($p < .001$). These somewhat reduced coefficients may reflect variability in performance associated with aging, with individuals with DS expected to show declines at relatively earlier chronological ages. We then selected only those individuals with ID with unspecified etiologies who were younger than 60 years of age ($N = 33$) and, therefore, were not expected to show declines in performance associated with normal aging, and found a Pearson correlation coefficient of

0.683 for the Total Score ($p < .001$) and a coefficient of 0.641 for the Free Recall Score ($p = .001$). These correlation coefficients indicate an acceptable level of comparability between the two versions of the Cued Recall Test.

Reliability of Retesting with the Same Test Version

Test–retest reliability was examined by comparing test scores of the same version separated by an interval of 3 years. When all healthy participants were included, the Pearson correlation coefficient was 0.390 for the Total Score ($p = .001$) and 0.388 for the Free Recall Score ($p = .002$). These scores are influenced, in part, by the longer interval between the administrations of the tests when the amount of decline may be amplified and when decline may be occurring at a faster rate in some individuals. Among individuals with ID from unspecified etiologies the coefficient for the Total Score increased to 0.428 but was not significant due to the reduced number of participants; the coefficient for the Free Recall Score of 0.623, however, was significant ($p = .002$). Overall, the Cued Recall Test appears to have modest test–retest reliability. A better measure of reliability would be to conduct repeated testing across different versions just days apart with a large sample, but this has yet to be done.

Diagnostic Efficacy

In the initial evaluation of our version of the Cued Recall Test there were 19 individ-uals with DS who had a diagnosis of DAD.[13] Based on their performance on this test, in comparison to that of their healthy peers with DS, our data sug-gested that a cutoff Total Score of ≤23 distinguished between the two groups. This cutoff score, however, reflected the performance characteristics of this specific group of participants. Since the publication of these findings, an additional 13 individuals have developed and received a diagnosis of dementia. For this new group of individuals we employed the same criteria for establishing the date of onset of DAD as previously; that is, the date of a physician's diagnosis. We then examined performance on the Cued Recall Test and found that the cutoff score of Total Score ≤ 23 identified all individuals with a diagnosis of DAD in this new group. In fact, the age at which 11 of these individuals, who had received a diag-nosis of DAD, met the cutoff score preceded the age of diagnosis from 9 to 84 months ($X = 29.2$ months); in the remaining two individuals it was concurrent with the diagnosis. This prospective group contributes to the validity of our choice of the particular level of the cutoff score.

We then examined the relationship between age at performing at the level of the cutoff score and age at diagnosis of DAD among all our participants with DS

($N = 32$). Twenty-nine individuals with DAD met the cutoff score at the time of their diagnosis and their scores on the Cued Recall Test continued to show subsequent declines. Indeed, many of these individuals met the cutoff score even prior to receiving their diagnosis and on subsequent testing their Total Score typically remained less than 23, indicating that the cutoff score represents a threshold. Three out of the 32 individuals with dementia did not quite reach the cutoff score at the time they received a diagnosis (Total Scores ranged from 24 to 26) although their scores at the time of diagnosis represented a decline from a previous level and their Total Score just prior to their diagnosis was ≤ 23 (Fig. 9.2). In general, a decline in Total Score to ≤ 23 should be considered a significant memory impairment in adults with DS and mild or moderate ID.

Sensitivity and Specificity

Sensitivity refers to the ability of a diagnostic test to identify individuals who have the disease and is directly related to the level of the cutoff score. In the case of a memory test that has the potential to be used as a screening test, it is important to set the cutoff score at a level high enough that it will identify all individuals who are in need of a diagnostic evaluation. To determine sensitivity, we examined only adults with DS because in our sample we have only one individual with ID of unspecified etiology who had a diagnosis of dementia. To test the sensitivity of the Cued Recall Test employing the cutoff score of ≤ 23, we examined performance on this test at the time of the clinical diagnosis, that is, when individuals first met the criteria for DAD. Since DAD is characterized by progressive decline, anyone with a diagnosis will eventually show global cognitive impairment and poor performance on any test of memory or cognition. It was, therefore, important to evaluate the Cued Recall Test at a time when individuals first met diagnostic criteria. For all other participants in our longitudinal study we used their score at their most recent testing.

The first estimate of sensitivity compared the participants with the diagnosis of DAD to all our other participants with DS. Among the group of participants without a diagnosis, there were very likely some individuals in a preclinical phase of DAD.[35] While recognizing this, we were interested in determining how effective the Cued Recall Test was in identifying individuals with DAD. In this analysis, the Total Score on the Cued Recall Test had a sensitivity of 91%, indicating that it detected most of the individuals who had a diagnosis of DAD.

Specificity refers to the ability of a test to correctly identify individuals who are without the disease. High specificity for a test can contribute diagnostic information by assisting in ruling out the presence of a particular disease. The specificity of the Cued Recall Test among the participants with DS was 72%. This lower score reflects the inclusion of some individuals who have MCI.

Positive predictive value (PPV) refers to the likelihood that a positive test result will be correct and is a measure of the efficiency of the screening test.

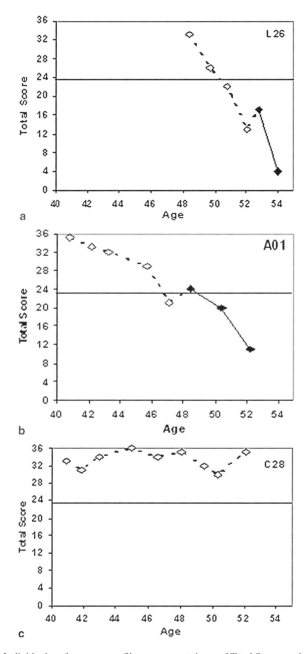

Fig. 9.2 (a–c) Individual performance profiles across test times of Total Score on the Cued Recall Test prior to (open circles) and after (closed circles) diagnosis of dementia. L26 met the cutoff score 3.2 years prior to a diagnosis and represents 83% of cases with dementia; A01 had a score close-to but not below the cutoff score at the time of diagnosis and represents 8.5% of cases. C28 has remained healthy

Predictive values are related to the prevalence of a condition or disease, with higher prevalence rates related to higher PPVs and lower negative predictive values (NPVs).[36] A comparison of all participants with and without a diagnosis gave a PPV of 58%. This score also reflects the inclusion of individuals with MCI who have memory impairment but who are for this analysis included in the nondemented group. A NPV refers to the likelihood that a person obtaining a score higher than the cutoff value is correctly identified as an individual without the disease. The NPV was 94%.

Mild Cognitive Impairment

Among our participants with DS there were 24 individuals who obtained a Total Score below the cutoff at the time of testing but did not have a diagnosis of DAD. For 22 of these individuals, we had longitudinal data that showed that their Total Score on the Cued Recall Test, at the most recent testing, represented a mean decline of 13.5 (SD = 8.5) points from the highest score they had received on previous testing. Their current performance, therefore, represented a change in their memory ability and can be correctly interpreted as memory impairment.

Fourteen individuals from the group with low scores on the Cued Recall Test also showed significant memory declines on a separate memory test, the SRT.[18,20] In a second analysis of the sensitivity of the Cued Recall Test we identified these 14 individuals as a group with MCI because there was independent verification of memory impairment but, since their skills of daily living were sufficiently preserved, they did not meet the criteria for a diagnosis of DAD. We compared their performance to individuals identified as "healthy," that is, participants without declines on the SRT (Table 9.2). In this analysis, sensitivity of the Cued Recall Test to identify individuals with MCI was 79% and the specificity was 84%; the PPV was 52% and the NPV was 94%. The lower PPV in this analysis may be due to the stringent criterion for significant memory decline on the SRT which has the effect of reducing the prevalence of individuals identified as having a "memory impairment."

Table 9.2 Comparison of Sensitivity, Specificity, Positive Predictive Value (PPV) and Negative Predictive Value (NPV) for Two and Three trials on the Cued Recall Test

Comparison	N	Sensitivity	Specificity	PPV	NPV
Three trials					
Demented vs nondemented	107	91	72	58	94
MCI vs healthy	75	79	84	52	94
Two trials					
Demented vs nondemented	107	91	69	56	95
MCI vs healthy	75	86	82	36	96

The cutoff score for two trials was a Total Score of ≤15 and for three trials was ≤23.

Longitudinal Data

We examined the longitudinal performance of ten individuals with a diagnosis of DAD for whom we had data for three complete test cycles across a time period from when they were thought to be healthy up to and after receiving their diagnosis. The interval we examined spanned a mean of 2.85 ± 7.3 years.[3] These individuals met the cutoff score on an average of 20 months (range = 0–39 months) prior to receiving a diagnosis of DAD. Two individuals (8.5%) met the cutoff score at the time of their diagnosis. The remaining two individuals (8.5%) did not meet the cutoff score at the time of their diagnosis although their scores were close (24 and 25) and their performance represented a decline from a previous level (see Fig. 9.2 for atypical profiles of performance).

The longitudinal analysis included scores from 48 individuals who were healthy (mean age = 44.9 ± 7.1 years; mean IQ = 53.4 ± 12.1), 9 with MCI (mean age = 51.6 ± 4.1 years; mean IQ = 50.7 ± 9.9), and 10 with a diagnosis of dementia (mean age = 53.4 ± 3.6 years; mean IQ = 54.1 ± 12.5). Analysis of covariance (ANCOVA) with Total Score across three test cycles as a repeated measure, with health status at the third cycle (healthy, MCI, dementia) as a between-subjects factor, and age and IQ as covariates showed a significant overall effect of health status ($F(1,62) = 57.528$, $p < .001$) that was modified by a health status × test cycle interaction ($F(4,122) = 8.509$, $p < .001$). While differences across test cycles in performance were not significantly related to age, there was an effect of IQ ($F(1,62) = 9.595$, $p < .01$) in which higher intelligence quotient (IQ) scores were, in general, associated with better performance on the test. Post hoc comparisons indicated that participants who were healthy had significantly better performance across test cycles than those with MCI ($F(1,53) = 53.808$, $p < .001$), but the difference between participants with MCI and those with DAD was not significant (Fig. 9.3).

In this longitudinal analysis, participants were categorized based on their health status at cycle 3. Within each of the groups, where individuals were classified as either MCI or demented, there is a pattern of decline that reflects their changing health status. In the group with MCI five of the nine individuals did not have memory impairment (defined as meeting the cutoff score) at cycle 1 and two did not have memory impairment at cycle 2. In the group with dementia, four of the ten individuals did not have memory impairment at cycle 1 but all had either MCI or dementia at cycle 2. The findings demonstrate a continuum of progressive memory impairment prior to and including the onset of dementia which was reflected in the Total Score of the Cued Recall Test. Further, these findings indicate that this test has good predictive validity.

---

[3] With the progression of DAD, some individuals became untestable and some individuals with and without dementia died over the course of this testing period, therefore, this analysis involved fewer individuals than the previously reported cross-sectional data.

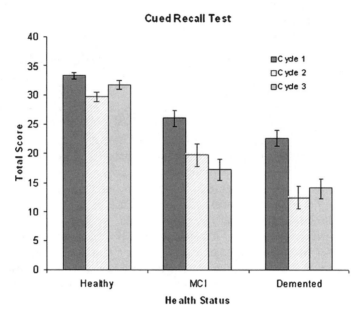

Cued Recall Test

Fig. 9.3 Means (with standard error bars) of longitudinal Total Scores on the Cued Recall Test for three groups of individuals with Down syndrome (DS). The healthy group is not suspected of decline, the group with Mild Cognitive Impairment (MCI) has significant memory declines on the Selective Reminding Test, and the group with dementia has a diagnosis of Alzheimer's disease

Normal Aging and Free Recall

Thus far we have discussed the role of the Total Score in identifying memory impairment associated with the preclinical and early-stage dementia. The Cued Recall Test also measures free recall and we first examined performance on this component in relation to age-associated changes in memory among those participants who have remained healthy and are not suspected of declines in functioning. An ANCOVA examined the Free Recall Score with etiology (DS, ID of unspecified etiology) as a between-subjects factor and age and IQ as covariates. Although adults with DS were poorer on Free Recall ($X = 12.73$, SD = 8.35) than adults with ID from unspecified etiologies ($X = 18.67$, SD = 9.16), this difference did not reach significance. There was a main effect of age ($F(1,117) = 19.43$, $p < .001$) that was modified by an etiology ×x age interaction ($F(1,117) = 6.36$, $p = .01$). Post hoc analysis of this interaction revealed age-associated declines on this memory measure for adults with DS ($F(2,58) = 12.61$, $p < .001$), but not for those with ID from unspecified etiologies.

Next, we examined whether the Free Recall component can distinguish between the groups with and without memory impairment among the adults with DS. We found that, once again, there were significant main effects of age ($F(1,102) = 20.01$, $p < .001$), IQ ($F(1,102) = 5.42$, $p = .02$), and health status ($F(1,102) = 20.35$,

$p < .001$). Post hoc analysis indicated that the healthy group was significantly different from both the MCI and dementia groups, but the latter two groups did not differ from one another.

These findings of performance on the Free Recall component essentially correspond to those of the Total Score. However, the Free Recall Scores have sufficient overlap across health status groups that it was difficult to determine an effective cutoff score with this measure.

Evaluation of Two Trials

In an effort to reduce the testing time for the Cued Recall Test, we examined our data to determine if we could achieve the same discrimination among the groups using scores from only the first two trials. We repeated the ANCOVA among the participants with DS with health status (healthy, MCI, demented) as a between-subjects factor and age and IQ as covariates employing a Total Score cutoff of ≤ 15 (out of a possible 24) and found a significant main effect of health status ($F(2,102) = 51.860$, $p < .001$). Once again there were significant effects for age ($F(1,102) = 7.793$, $p = .006$) with older participants having poorer scores, and IQ ($F(1,102) = 14.921$, $p < .001$) with lower IQ scores associated with poorer scores. Post hoc analysis showed that healthy participants performed significantly better than either the group with MCI or dementia.

We repeated the calculations for sensitivity and specificity (Table 9.2) and found that a cutoff Total Score of ≤ 15 for only two trials was adequate to discriminate between individuals who were demented from the group that was not demented (healthy and MCI) and also between individuals who had MCI from those who were healthy. The PPV, however, reflected the relatively high number of false positives with the cutoff score of ≤ 15.

Pros and Cons of Cued Recall Test

The Cued Recall Test is appropriate for the evaluation of adults with developmental disabilities in the mild to moderate range of ID. Verbal ability is required but, in our experience, some individuals with a receptive vocabulary as low as an age equivalent of 2.5 years (as measured by the Peabody Picture Vocabulary Test—Revised[37]) have successfully performed on the Cued Recall Test. The principal advantage of this test is its ability to distinguish between individuals who have significant memory impairment from those who are healthy. Further, the test appears to be sensitive to the memory impairment that precedes the onset of the symptoms that are the basis for a diagnosis of dementia (DSM-IV[38]; ICD-10[39]). In fact, the cutoff score identifies most individuals with MCI. Early diagnosis is useful in planning for individuals and, when treatment becomes available, it will be essential.

More importantly, this test has the potential to be a useful screening tool because of its ability to identify memory impairment at a single evaluation. If the overall level-of-functioning of an individual can be established to be within the mild to moderate range of ID then the Total Score on the Cued Recall Test can be interpreted without reference to a baseline score. The ability of this test to detect memory impairment may facilitate an earlier diagnosis of dementia because the score indicating "memory impairment" is not based on an interval of documented decline.

Ideally, however, adults would be administered this test while they are healthy to establish a baseline of their performance, and then would be periodically retested. Systematic, longitudinal assessments would firmly establish a decline in memory ability. For adults with DS, the suggested age for a baseline test administration is 40 years, with retests every 3 years.

The three-trial version of the Cued Recall Test requires about 20 min to complete and should be administered by an Examiner familiar with testing procedures, in general, and with testing individuals with intellectual impairment, in particular. Our findings indicate that a cutoff score based on the three trials is efficacious. However, a preliminary analysis showed that two trials may be sufficient, but this needs to be confirmed with prospective data.

With respect to the specific value of the cutoff score, we set it at a Total Score of ≤23 for three trials based on our longitudinal study. At this time, the Cued Recall Test has been used only in the context of research and by only one laboratory. The participants in the longitudinal study have been tested repeatedly over a number of years and are familiar with the Examiners and the testing procedures. This may have biased their performance in the direction of better scores. When this test is used by investigators who are assessing individuals for the first time, the cutoff score may need to be set at a slightly lower level in order to identify memory impairment.

On the other hand, if the Cued Recall Test is employed as a screening tool for identifying individuals who need a clinical evaluation, then a somewhat higher cutoff score might be needed. In our sample, a cutoff score of ≤26 would have identified all individuals with a diagnosis of DAD (but would have increased the false-positive rate, also). An optimum cutoff score will be determined, in the future, when the Cued Recall Test is employed by investigators in diverse settings. It may be that a conservative cutoff score would be of more use for researchers, while a more liberal value would be more useful in clinical screening programs.

While the strength of our longitudinal study has been an ability to follow, carefully, adults with DS over an extended period of time, the study has a relatively small number of individuals. In the current analysis, we applied a criterion we previously established to a new group of individuals who were showing declines and found it to be applicable. Future studies will broaden the data base to include individuals from a variety of contexts, including clinical settings, and individuals with various etiologies.

Studies comparing scores from different testers and test versions, and test–retest on the same version, will also be needed in order to rigorously determine reliability.

Our longitudinal studies have shown that even healthy individuals have small variations in performance on this test (see performance of participant C28 in Fig. 9.1). Reliability studies will be useful in interpreting individual variability. However, even without these reliability studies in hand, the Cued Recall Test appears to be able to assign adults with DS and mild or moderate ID to the categories of either memory impaired or memory unimpaired.

The Cued Recall Test is not useful for individuals with few or no verbal abilities nor is it applicable to individuals with IQs below 30. In addition, we have evaluated only individuals with DS and, therefore, do not know if the criterion we have established is appropriate for individuals with ID from other etiologies.

Summary

Findings from our study employing the Cued Recall Test indicate that individuals with even very early-stage DAD are unlikely to achieve a Total Score greater than 23. Having a test with a cutoff score will be very useful to assessment protocols whereby memory impairment can be established at a single evaluation. Although there was variability in performance across test cycles that reduced reliability assessments, healthy participants, in general, maintained scores above the cutoff score. We were also able to demonstrate that individuals who received a diagnosis of DAD had a history of decline in memory performance on this test.

Individuals with MCI and individuals with early-stage DAD had significant memory impairment and were distinguished from the healthy participants by their performance on Total Scores on the Cued Recall Test. To distinguish between an individual with MCI and an individual with early-stage DAD, evidence is needed of cognitive and functional decline on additional measures.

The Cued Recall Test will be a useful component of a screening test battery for older adults with DS. It is relatively easy and quick to administer, is noninvasive, and it identifies most individuals who are in need of further evaluation for DAD. Further, it identifies individuals in an early stage of memory decline at a time when intervention would be most beneficial.

Acknowledgments The authors would like to thank Phyllis Kittler, Ph.D. and Catherine Marino, R.N. for their many contributions to this longitudinal study. We are grateful to the participants and their families for their cooperation and the agencies that have supported us and extended their hospitality during our test sessions: AHRC New York League Workshops in Manhattan and the Bronx; ARC of Westchester; ARC of New Jersey; Brooklyn Guild for Exceptional Children and the Conklin Residence; Builders of Family and Youth of the Diocese of Brooklyn; Pathfinder Village; and Wassaic Developmental Center. We also thank all diagnosticians who shared their findings with us. In particular we would like to acknowledge the contributions of Dr. J. Tsouris, Dr. Madrid, and P. Patti, M.A. from the George Jervis Clinic of the NYS Institute for Basic Research. Finally, we would like to thank Dr. Ausma Rabe and Dr. Ira Cohen for critical comments on the manuscript. This work has been supported by funds from the New York State Office of Mental Retardation and Developmental Disabilities and NIH grants PO1 AG 11531 to H.M. Wisniewski, PO1 HD35897 to W. Silverman and RO1 AG 14771 to D.A. Devenny.

References

1. Brown LB and Storandt M (2000) Sensitivity of category cued recall to very mild dementia of the Alzheimer type. Arch Clin Neuropsychol 15:529–34.
2. Petersen RC, Smith GE, Ivnik RJ, et al. (1994) Memory function in very early Alzheimer's disease. Neurology 44:867–72.
3. Devenny DA, Krinsky-McHale SJ, Sersen G, et al. (2000) Sequence of cognitive decline in dementia in adults with Down's syndrome. J Intellect Disabil Res 44:654–65.
4. Hawkins BA, Eklund SJ, James DR, et al. (2003) Adaptive behavior and cognitive function of adults with Down syndrome: Modeling change with age. Ment Retard 41:7–28.
5. Oliver C, Crayton L, Holland A, et al. (1998) A four year prospective study of age-related cognitive change in adults with Down's syndrome. Psychol Med 28:1365–77.
6. Grober E, Buschke H, Crystal H, et al. (1988) Screening for dementia by memory testing. Neurology 38:900–3.
7. Craik FIM, Byrd M, and Swanson JM (1987) Patterns of memory loss in three elderly samples. Psychol Aging 2:79–86.
8. Buschke H, Sliwinski MJ, Kuslansky G, et al. (1997) Diagnosis of early dementia by the Double Memory Test: Encoding specificity improves diagnostic sensitivity and specificity. Neurology 48:989–97.
9. Grober E and Kawas C (1997) Learning and retention in preclinical and early Alzheimer's disease. Psychol Aging 12:183–8.
10. Grober E, Lipton RB, Katz M, et al. (1998) Demographic influences on free and cued selective reminding performance in older persons. J Clin Exp Neuropsychol 20:221–6.
11. Ivanoiu A, Adam S, van der Linden M, et al. (2005) Memory evaluation with a new cued recall test in patients with mild cognitive impairment and Alzheimer's disease. J Neurol 252:47–55.
12. Tuokko H, Vernon-Wilkinson R, Weir J, et al. (1991) Cued recall and early identification of dementia. J Clin Exp Neuropsychol 13:871–9.
13. Devenny DA, Zimmerli EJ, Kittler P, et al. (2002) Cued recall in early-stage dementia in adults with Down's syndrome. J Intellect Disabil Res 46:472–83.
14. Grober E and Buschke H (1987) Genuine memory deficits in dementia. Dev Neuropsychol 3:13–36.
15. Tulving E (2002) Episodic memory: From mind to brain. Annu Rev Psychol 53:1–25.
16. Lepage M, Ghaffar O, Nyberg L, et al. (2000) Prefrontal cortex and episodic memory retrieval mode. Proc Natl Acad Sci 97:506–11.
17. Holland AJ, Hon J, Huppert FA, et al. (2000) Incidence and course of dementia in people with Down's syndrome: Findings from a population-based study. J Intellect Disabil Res 44:138–46.
18. Devenny DA, Silverman WP, Hill AL, et al. (1996) Normal ageing in adults with Down's syndrome: A longitudinal study. J Intellect Disabil Res 40:208–21.
19. Haxby JV and Schapiro MB (1992) Longitudinal study of neuropsychological function in older adults with Down syndrome. Prog Clin Biol Res 379:35–50.
20. Krinsky-McHale SJ, Devenny DA, and Silverman WP (2002) Changes in explicit memory associated with early dementia in adults with Down's syndrome. J Intellect Disabil Res 46:198–208.
21. Dalton AJ, Mehta PD, Fedor BL, et al. (1999) Cognitive changes in memory precede those in praxis in aging persons with Down syndrome. J Intellect Dev Disabil 24:169–87.
22. Devenny DA, Krinsky-McHale SJ, and Kittler P (1999) Age-associated changes in modality preference in adults with Down syndrome. In: 32nd Annual Gatlinburg Conference on Research and Theory in Mental Retardation and Developmental Disabilities, Charleston, SC, 1999.
23. Devenny DA, Kittler P, and Krinsky-McHale SJ (2007) Declines in visuo-spatial abilities in young adults with Down syndrome. In: 40th Annual Gatlinburg conference on Research and Theory in Intellectual & Developmental Disabilities, Annapolis, MD, 2007, p. 84.

24. Huppert FA (1994) Memory function in dementia and normal aging—dimensions or dichotomy? In: Huppert FA, Brayne C, and O'Connor DW, eds. Dementia and Normal Aging. Cambridge, UK: Cambridge University Press, pp. 291–330.
25. Petersen RC, Doody R, Kurz A, et al. (2001) Current concepts in mild cognitive impairment. Arch Neurol 58:1985–92.
26. Petersen RC, Stevens JC, Ganguli M, et al. (2001) Practice parameter: Early detection of dementia: Mild cognitive impairment (an evidence based review). Report of the Quality Standards Subcommittee of the American Academy of Neurology. Neurology 56:1133–42.
27. Elias MF, Beiser A, Wolf PA, et al. (2000) The preclinical phase of Alzheimer disease: A 22-year prospective study of the Framingham Cohort. Arch Neurol 57:808–13.
28. Flicker C, Ferris SH, and Reisberg B (1991) Mild cognitive impairment in the elderly: Predictors of dementia. Neurology 41:1006–9.
29. Morris JC, Storandt M, Miller P, et al. (2001) Mild cognitive impairment represents early-stage Alzheimer disease. Arch Neurol 58:397–405.
30. Petersen RC, Smith GE, Waring SC, et al. (1999) Mild cognitive impairment: Clinical characterization and outcome. Arch Neurol 56:303–8.
31. Bozoki A, Giordani B, Heidebrink JL, et al. (2001) Mild cognitive impairments predict dementia in nondemented elderly patients with memory loss. Arch Neurol 58:411–6.
32. Small BJ, Fratiglioni L, Viitanen M, et al. (2000) The course of cognitive impairment in preclinical Alzheimer disease: Three- and 6-year follow-up of a population-based sample. Arch Neurol 57:839–44.
33. Buschke H (1984) Cued recall in amnesia. J Clin Neuropsychol 6:433–40.
34. Snodgrass JG and Vanderward M (1980) A standardized set of 260 pictures: Norms for naming agreement, familiarity, and visual complexity. J Exp Psychol: Human Learn Memory 6:174–215.
35. Sliwinski MJ, Hofer SM, Hall C, et al. (2003) Modeling memory decline in older adults: the importance of preclinical dementia, attention and chronological age. Psychol Aging 18:658–71.
36. Loong T (2005) Understanding sensitivity and specificity with the right side of the brain. BMJ 327:716–9.
37. Dunn LM and Dunn LM (1981) Peabody Picture Vocabulary Test—Revised. Circle Pines, MN: American Guidance Service.
38. American Psychiatric Association (1994) Diagnostic and Statistical Manual of Mental Disorders, 4th edn. Washington, DC: American Psychiatric Association.
39. World Health Organization (1992) ICD-10: International Statistical Classification of Diseases and Related Health Problems, 10th edn. Geneva: World Health Organization.

Chapter 10
The Adaptive Behavior Dementia Questionnaire (ABDQ)

V.P. Prasher

Introduction

The concept of adaptive behavior has been defined by Heber in 1961[1] as "the effectiveness with which the individual copes with the nature and social demands of this environment" and by Gunzberg in 1977[2] as "the extent to which an individual is able and willing to conform to the customs, habits and standards of behavior prevailing in the society in which he lives; by the degree to which he is able to do so independently of direction and guidance and by the extent to which he participates constructively in the affairs and conduct of his community." Adaptive behavior scales (ABSs) assess an individual's current abilities as they are manifested in a given situation. Several measures and patterns of behavior are assessed in different situations to give an overall assessment. Individual items are grouped together into domains. Such domains include, for example, communication, dressing, feeding, and toileting.

Background

Zigman and colleagues in Chapter 6 give a full and detailed review of the role of adaptive behavior in the assessment of dementia in persons with intellectual disability (ID). This chapter will focus specifically on the *AAMR Adaptive Behavior Scale* (ABS)[3] and how it was used to develop the Adaptive Behavior Dementia Questionnaire (ABDQ).

Several studies have recently been published investigating the assessment of adaptive behavior in persons with ID (Table 10.1). The majority of studies have used the ABS as the measure of choice. It is designed to provide objective descriptions and evaluations of an individual's behavior in coping with the natural and social demands of his/her environment. The ABS consists of two parts. Part I (independent functioning) is designed to evaluate an individual's skills and habits in ten behavior domains considered important to the development of personal independence in daily living. The 10 behavior domains and 21 subdomains are given in

V.P. Prasher (ed.), *Neuropsychological Assessments of Dementia in Down Syndrome and Intellectual Disabilities,*
DOI: 10.1007/978-1-84800-249-4_10, © Springer Science+Business Media, LLC 2009

Table 10.1 Recent Reports Investigating Adaptive behavior in the Intellectually Disabled Population

Authors	Sample (population)	Age-range (years)	Residence	Main findings
Schupf and colleagues[4]	99 DS individuals 99 non-ID individuals DS and ID controls)	20–69	Institution community	DS adults over 50 had significant greater regression than controls and younger DS individuals during the last 3 years of life
Brown and colleagues[5]	130 (DS)	1–59	Institution community	Age-related decline present. Least decline for individuals resident in institutional settings
Rasmussen and Sobsey[6]	56 DS individuals 64 ID individuals (DS and ID)	–	Institution	Decline in skills for individuals over 40 years of age. Particularly in self-help and communication skills. Adaptive skills more stable for ID groups
Burt and colleagues[7]	34 (DS)	22–56	Community	No age-related decline in nondemented middle-aged DS individuals. Level of ID significant factor in analysis
Roeden and Zitman[8]	115 (DS and ID)	31–62	Community	Loss of skills in adults with DS >50 years. Dementia factor in loss. Nonsignificant loss due to visual decline
Prasher et al.[9]	128 (DS)	16–72	Institution community	Decline in skills for middle-aged DS population over 3-year period of assessment. Only one significant factor for decline dementia

DS, Down syndrome; ID, intellectually disabled.

Table 10.2. Part II (maladaptive behaviors) of the scale is designed to provide measures of maladaptive behavior related to personality and behavior disorders. Part II consists of 14 domains (Table 10.3).

The scale is completed by a person familiar with the person with ID or by a semi-interview assessment with the interviewer filling out the scale item-by-item while obtaining information from the person familiar with the subject. In the latter case it is possible to clarify and extend the questioning about individual items. The ABS is one of the most widely used and best standardized instruments and has been shown to have good reliability and validity.[10–12]

A number of researchers have previously used the ABS to assess age-related changes in adults with DS (Table 10.4).

Table 10.2 Adaptive Behavior Scale Part I Domains

I. Independent functioning
  A. Eating
  B. Toilet use
  C. Cleanliness
  D. Appearance
  E. Care of clothing
  F. Dressing and undressing
  G. Travel
  H. Independent functioning
II. Physical development
  A. Sensory development
  B. Motor development
III. Economic activity
  A. Money handling
  B. Shopping skills
IV. Language development
  A. Expression
  B. Comprehension
  C. Social language
V. Numbers and time
VI. Domestic activity
  A. Cleaning
  B. Kitchen duties
  C. Domestic activities
VII. Vocational activity
VIII. Self-direction
  A. Initiative
  B. Perseverance
  C. Leisure time
IX. Responsibility
X. Socialization

Table 10.3 Adaptive Behavior Scale Part II Domains

I. Violent and destructive behavior
II. Antisocial behavior
III. Rebellious behavior
IV. Untrustworthy behavior
V. Withdrawal
VI. Stereotyped behavior and odd mannerisms
VII. Inappropriate interpersonal manners
VIII. Unacceptable vocal habits
IX. Unacceptable or eccentric habits
X. Self-abusive behavior
XI. Hyperactive tendencies
XII. Sexually aberrant behavior
XIII. Psychological disturbances
XIV. Use of medications

Table 10.4 Principal Studies Using the ABS to Assess Aging in Persons with Down Syndrome

Authors	Sample (population)	Age (years)	Residence	Main findings
Miniszek[13]	19	34+	–	Older (>50 years) DS persons scored lower on the ABS than younger (<50 years) persons. Regressed persons scored significantly lower than nonregressed controls
Collacott[14]	308	18+	Institution community	Age-related exponential decline
Prasher and Chung[15]	201	16+	Institution community	Age-related decline found. Significant causative factors were aging, severity of ID, and presence of DAD. Absence of a medical illness was a predictor of higher scores
Collacott[16]	351	18+	Institution community	DS persons with late-onset seizures had lower adaptive scores than older control group and the early-onset seizure DS group
Prasher and colleagues[9]	128	16–72	Institution community	Decline in skills for middle-aged DS population over 3-year period of assessment. Only one significant factor for decline dementia
Prasher[17]	57	17–71	Institution community	Significant decline in ABS scores over 5-year period for persons with dementia as compared with controls

Miniszek[13] was able to show that elderly persons with DS ($N = 15$, age >50 years) scored lower on the ABS than did younger DS ($N = 4$ age <50 years) subjects in every area of adaptive functioning except in domestic functioning. The elderly DS group was divided into nine residents, judged to be severely regressed, and six who were still functioning relatively well. The regressed group scored much lower in all areas. An individual subject could, on comparison of their ABS profile with the above profiles, be reasonably diagnosed as having regression and dementia if other causes of regression were excluded.

Collacott[14] examined age-related changes of adaptive behavior in 308 adults with DS who were identified through the Leicestershire Mental Handicap Register. Scores for each domain of ABS Part I were analyzed for each age-related cohort. Mean scores for older subjects (>30 years) were compared to those below this age. Collacott found a significant reduction within the domain of physical development (which included sensory impairment and locomotor disability) for the cohort aged 40–49 years. For those in the age cohort 50–59, deterioration occurred in all domains. Statistical significance was found for the domains of physical development, economic activity, numeracy and time sense, domestic activities, and vocational activities. After the age of 60 years, significant deterioration occurred in all domains. No consistent age-related changes were found for maladaptive behavior.

For the total population decline with age followed an algebraic curve in which the overall ABS score was a function of the square of the individual's age.

Prasher and colleagues[9,15,17] in a number of articles investigating changes in adaptive behavior in 201 adults with DS over a 5-year period confirmed the association between decline in adaptive skills and aging and dementia in older adults with DS. The researchers were able to specifically correlate decline in ABS scores with onset and deterioration in dementia in Alzheimer's disease (DAD). Particular domains of ABS Part I, which showed significant change, were independent functioning, numbers and time, self-direction, and responsibility.

Following research over a period of 20 years, using the ABS to assess change in adaptive behavior in older adults with DS it was apparent that the ABS could be used as a neuropsychological measure to detect and monitor DAD in adults with DS. Particular domains of ABS Part I were, therefore, used to device a questionnaire to screen for DAD in adults with DS. This is described below.

Development of the ABDQ

Sample Group

One-hundred and fifty adults with DS, living in the same geographical region, were recruited. Baseline demographic data of age, gender, karyotyping for DS, residence, and severity of ID were available. Severity of premorbid ID was assessed by (1) review of previously reported intelligence tests, (2) previous level of functioning as determined by review of medical notes, from carer interview and from the mental state examination of the individual. Severity of ID was classified using ICD-10 criteria.[18]

Of the 150 adults with DS who participated, 83 (55%) were male and 67 (45%) were female. The mean age of the sample at the start of the assessments was 44.0 years (SD 11.46; range 16–76 years). All individuals had physical stigmata of DS with 92% trisomy 21 (of 135 tested) and 6% of those tested had translocated form of DS. Sixty (40%) were resident in their family home, 57 (38%) in community group homes, and 33 (22%) resided in the hospital. Twenty-seven (18%) individuals had mild ID, 104 (69%) moderate, and 19 (13%) severe ID.

Assessments

All persons were being followed up on an annual basis as part of ongoing clinical care with detailed reassessments of their physical and mental health, adaptive behavior, and social needs. Carers and individuals were interviewed to elicit any evidence of any significant medical condition. As part of the care provision

individuals underwent annual (where compliant) venepuncture for routine hemato-
logical (including B_{12} and folate levels), biochemical (including plasma glucose),
and thyroid screening. Brain magnetic resonance imaging was also undertaken in a
number of cases. Psychiatric assessments were undertaken by using Part 1 Section
H of the Cambridge Mental Disorders of the Elderly Examination (CAMDEX)
schedule,[19] standard mental state examination of individuals, and completion of
the ICD-10 Symptom Checklist for Mental Disorders.[20] As recommended by the
international research community[21] all available information was reviewed annually to determine the presence of mental disorder according to ICD-10 criteria, and
in particular DAD.[18] Adaptive functioning of the individuals was assessed annually
for five consecutive years using the ABS.[3]

Findings for the absence or presence of DAD were compared to change in the
ABS measurements over the 5-year collection period to determine which items of
the ABS best correlated with deterioration in intellectual functioning and could be
subsequently used to develop a screening questionnaire.

Development of Questionnaire

In order to diagnose DAD there must be evidence of decline in any given criteria.
For this reason the differences in the ABS scores across the 5-year period were
analyzed to see if any pattern emerged. The differences that were examined were
those of the scores obtained in year 1 subtracted from those of years 2, 3, 4, and 5.
Hence a decline in any area was reflected by a negative difference. To compare the
ABS findings with the diagnosis of DAD, a new variable called "DCHANGEi"
(where i = year 2, 3, 4, or 5) was introduced. This variable took 1 or 2 possible
values and these were assigned as in Table 10.5.

Only patients who were nondemented at the beginning of the 5-year period and
were still alive after the data collection period participated in the subsequent data
analysis. Four adults died by year 3, 11 died by year 4, and 19 persons died during
the 5-year period. This part of the analysis looked at the change in the DAD state,
i.e., comparing those that remained nondemented over the 5-year data collection
period ($N = 103$) to those who were initially nondemented but were diagnosed with
DAD ($N = 16$) at some point in the time period. This diagnosis of DAD was independent to information obtained from the ABS data.

In order to get a spread of items from all Part I, ten domains of the ABS, each
domain was analyzed individually to see which of the items in each domain were

Table 10.5 Scoring Criteria for DCHANGEi

Is the patient demented in year 1?	Is the patient demented in year i?	DCHANGEi
No	No	0
No	Yes	1

the best at predicting the onset of DAD. The analysis to find the best predictors was performed by using two primary methods of analysis, logistic regression analysis and stepwise discriminant analysis.

Identification of Significant ABS Items

Using logistic regression analysis, individual items of the 66 items of Part I of the ABS which produced significant results for a particular time period were identified. For example for domain I, items 3 and 42 (drinking and time, respectively) were significant when the difference in the scores obtained over the time period covering years 1 to 2 was considered. Thirty-one items appeared to be predictors for the onset of DAD. It was attempted to remove the least possible items from the questionnaire to make it less parsimonious but at the same time obtaining some useful results with the logistic regression analysis. After examining correlations between the 31 items, it was possible to reduce further the number to 16 items. Therefore, the 16 Part I ABS items whose change was shown to differentiate individuals with DS who develop DAD from those who do not were:

1. Tooth brushing
2. Dressing
3. Control of hands
4. Purchasing
5. Conversation
6. Time
7. Food preparation
8. Table clearing
9. Job complexity
10. Job performance
11. Initiative
12. Persistence
13. Personal belongings
14. Cooperation
15. Participation in group activities
16. Social maturity

To confirm that changes in the final 16 ABS items were of clinical significance, logistic regression analysis on these items with DCHANGE5 as the response and the items above as the model was performed. The model also included the patient's age, sex, place of residence, and severity of ID, as there was reason to believe these factors would have an effect on the outcome.

If the differences over the 5-year time period are considered, a list of each individual's probability of getting DAD over the 5 years can be obtained. The descriptive statistics for this is given in Table 10.6, split according to DCHANGE5.

Table 10.6 Descriptive Statistics for Each Individual Getting DAD Over the 5-Year Period

Variable DCHANGE5	Number	Mean	Median	Standard deviation	SE Mean
Probability 0	103	0.03044	0.00002	0.08127	0.00801
1	16	0.8040	0.8657	0.2548	0.0637

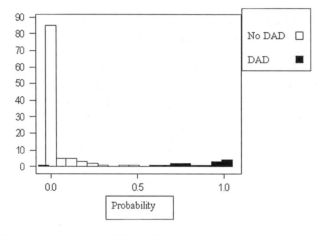

Fig. 10.1 Histogram showing probabilities of dementia computed using the 16 ABS items

Figure 10.1 shows the probabilities, split according to DCHANGE5. A clear distinction between the probabilities for the nondemented (white bars) and those that are diagnosed with DAD (black bars) over the 5-year time period are evident. This finding is also emphasized when considering the sensitivity ($15/16 = 94\%$) and specificity ($88/103 = 85\%$) of the questionnaire. These are both very high when a cutoff probability of 0.5 is used indicating an accurate test.

Composing the Questionnaire

Identification of change in 16 items of the Part I of the ABS had been shown above to be good predictors for the development of DAD in adults with DS. The 16 items were now compiled into a questionnaire format that focussed on decline in these 16 items over time. Each item consisted of a question asking whether the respondent had recently experienced a change in a particular behavior on a scale ranging from "better than normal" to "much worse than normal" (where "normal" referred to when the respondent was well and before the onset of any recent ill-health). Errors due to "tendency to agree" were reduced by avoiding the use of a bimodal response scale and "error of central tendency" was eliminated by having an even number of response categories. The four-point response scale was treated as a multiple-response scale (Likert scale) with scores of 0, 1, 2, and 3 assigned to the four positions.

Calibration of the questionnaire was undertaken using two calibration groups—DS adults who were well, and those who had a clinical diagnosis of DAD according to ICD-10 criteria.[18] The latter group consisted of mildly demented, moderately demented, and severely demented persons. This approach was necessary to save items which could discriminate people who were well from those with mild DAD but at the same time be sensitive to various degrees of severity of DAD.

The questionnaire was sent out to a further sample of 100 DS individuals, with targeting to those DS persons with DAD, selected from those known to the clinical service. This sample included individuals were had not participated in the initial part of the study. Seventy-four completed questionnaires were returned (48 from non-DAD persons and 26 from patients with DAD). Each questionnaire was completed by the principal carer (family or paid carer). For those individuals who were also cared for by a second carer who also knew the patient in question well, the second carer was asked to complete and return the questionnaire independently of the first carer. Forty-two questionnaires were sent to a second carer, of which 36 were returned.

Questionnaire Analysis

It was apparent after the tests were returned that a significant proportion of carers had difficulty in answering the first question "Are they able to brush their teeth?" If the person had no teeth then "decline" in this behavior was not possible. Since approximately 15% of the returns had difficulty in completing this question, it was decided that this question would be excluded from any subsequent analysis, leaving 15 questions.

The final 15 questions of the ABDQ are given in Appendix 8.

The responses were coded as 0 (better than normal), 1 (same as normal), 2 (worse than normal), and 3 (much worse than normal). Analysis using the total of the 15 items was initially undertaken but improvement was found if a weighted total of the 15 items was used. A suitable weighting was derived as follows.

A series of 16 logistic regressions were performed each using two independent variables; the total of the 15 items and an individual item score. The most significant individual item was then identified and its weighting varied in the total score in line with its coefficient in the corresponding logistic regression. With this new "total" the above process was repeated until the weighting of each item had been reviewed. The weightings finally derived are shown in Table 10.7.

Figure 10.2 illustrates dot plots that show the total weighted score (TWS) obtained by the patients split according to DAD status using the ABDQ questionnaire. They show a clear distinction between the scores obtained by the

Table 10.7 Weightings for Questions in Questionnaire

Question	Item	Weighting
1	Are they able to dress themselves better/same/worse than normal?	1
2	Can they use their hands better/same/worse than normal?	4
3	Is their ability to buy/shop better/same/worse than normal?	1
4	Are they able to have a conversation better/same/worse than normal?	1
5	Is their awareness of time better/same/worse than normal?	4
6	Do they help to prepare food better/same/worse than normal?	1
7	Do they help to clear the table better/same/worse than normal?	6
8	Are they able to perform simple jobs better/same/worse than normal?	4
9	Do they carry out simple jobs better/same/worse than normal?	5
10	Is their initiative in doing activities better/same/worse than normal?	1
11	Is their persistence in doing activities better/same/worse than normal?	1
12	Do they take care of their personal belongings better/same/worse than normal?	3
13	Is their cooperation better/same/worse than normal?	3
14	Do they participate in group activities better/same/worse than normal?	1
15	Is their ability to do things independently better/same/worse than normal?	1

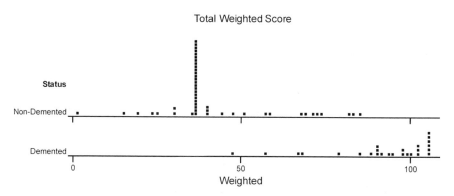

Fig. 10.2 Dot plot for demented versus nondemented DS individuals

nondemented and demented patient. Using a cutoff score on the TWS of greater than 78, a sensitivity for the ABDQ questionnaire to detect DAD was 89% and a specificity of 94%. The positive predictive value was 89% and the negative predictive value was 94%. The overall percentage correct identification (accuracy) of DAD and non-DAD cases was 92%.

Using the weighted items the questionnaire was developed further to categorize individuals into non-DAD mild DAD, moderate DAD, and severe DAD. The cutoff scores for the ABDQ for an ordinal logistic regression with severity of DAD according to ICD-10 criteria[18] and the weighted totals of the 15 items are given in Table 10.8.

Table 10.8 Questionnaire Cutoff Scores for Severity of DAD

Severity of DAD[a]	Cutoff scores of ABDQ
No dementia in Alzheimer's disease	< 78
Mild dementia in Alzheimer's disease	78–89
Moderate dementia in Alzheimer's disease	90–99
Severe dementia in Alzheimer's disease	> = 100

[a] Dementia in Alzheimer's disease.

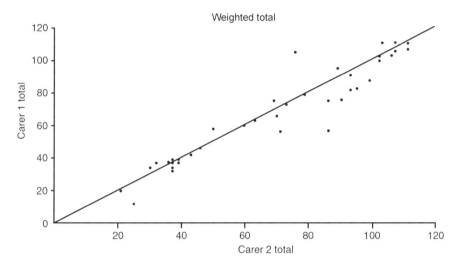

Fig. 10.3 ABDQ interrater reliability

Psychometric Properties of ABDQ

Interrater Reliability

The TWS from one carer was correlated with that reported by the second carer (N = 36) (see Fig. 10.3). Pearson correlation was 0.954 ($P < 0.01$). The findings demonstrate that the ABDQ questionnaire has good interrater reliability.

Validity

Face Validity

It has now been well established in the literature[22,23] that onset and deterioration of clinical AD in adults with DS is associated with a significant decline in adaptive behavior. Further the principle instrument that has been used to measure adaptive

behavior has been the ABS.[3] The items of the ABDQ questionnaire were derived
from the ABS[3] and therefore do have good face validity. The 15 selected items
which make up the ABDQ involve the detection of change in many of the different
areas of abilities which are known to be affected in DAD, e.g., in orientation to
time, attention, speech, self-care skills, social and occupational skills. Deterioration
in adaptive behavior can, therefore, reflect decline in intellectual, social behavior,
personal activities and emotional aspects of DAD.

Split-Half Validity

In order to verify the face validity, split-half validity was undertaken. To do this 74
patients were randomly split into two halves with 24 nondemented and 13 demented
patients in each half. One half was then used to derive a weighting as above and the
other half used to determine the validity of the weighted totals. All the items that
were found to have weightings >1 were those that had greater weighting previously.
There was good agreement between the two sets of results. The results of the binary
logistic regression using the new weighted items gave an overall accuracy of 94%,
and was comparable to 92% found previously.

Future Issues

Further field trials investigating the psychometric properties and clinical accuracy of
the ABDQ to detect DAD in adults with DS are recommended. However, readers
should be aware that the ABDQ has not been tested on non-DS adults with dementia,
in persons with deterioration in physical health or onset of non-DAD psychiatric
disorders, or investigated for the effects of demographic variables (e.g., age, race).
Researchers are encouraged to investigate the use of the ABDQ in these areas.

Summary

Previous research by the authors[9,22] over a 10-year period using the ABS[3] has
demonstrated that this instrument can significantly measure deterioration of DAD
in adults with DS. This work has led to the development of this questionnaire which
can be completed on all older adults with DS, irrespective of the underlying ID or
degree of test compliance, which is an informant-based questionnaire, which has
now been shown to have good reliability, validity, and accuracy. It is user-friendly
and takes approximately 10–15 min to complete.

There continues to be ongoing methodological issues on flaws relating to research
in the field of ID. The recruited sample size was 150 adults but was reduced to 119
persons for appropriate data analysis. However, this size remains a large sample compared to other previous studies in the field. This sample was found to be representative

of adults with DS as it included a wide age range, males and females, different degrees of severity of ID and individuals resident in different settings. A significant number of individuals were diagnosed as having DAD (44 individuals) during the period, and again although this number may appear small compared to studies in the non-ID population, it is relatively large for studies of people with ID.

The problem of a gold standard in the diagnosis of DAD is an ongoing issue. The diagnostic process used was that recommended by the international research community.[21] Further, in this study individuals diagnosed with DAD were followed up (up to 6 years) after the diagnosis was made which allowed the reliabi =lity of the diagnosis according to ICD-10 criteria[18] to be further validated. The diagnosis of DAD was independent of the adaptive behavior assessment, and the analysis of the ABS data only took place after the 5-year period, ensuring no cross-contamination of data. Individuals with other causes of dementia other than DAD were excluded as part of the diagnostic process for DAD, and therefore, these findings reflect the specific screening for DAD in adults with DS, and not just for a general dementia disorder.

The diagnosis of DAD in the ID population requires further research. At present no definitive antimortem measure is available, and although a number of other neuropsychological measures to screen for dementia have been developed, virtually none have been accepted internationally and are not designed to specifically detect DAD. The Dementia Questionnaire for Mentally Retarded Persons[24] is now widely used for screening for dementia. Conflicting results have been found regarding its validity[25,26] to detect DAD although it may prove to be of value as a tool to assess treatment response in drug trials.[27] Other measures such as the Dementia Scale for Down Syndrome[28] have been produced, but again their reliability and validity needs to be independently researched.[29] The ABDQ has been developed from over 10 years of research investigating changes in adaptive behavior in adults with Down syndrome. It can be used for all adults with ID, irrespective of the severity of ID or DAD. It is "user-friendly" and specifically screens for DAD not just dementia per se.

Acknowledgment   This chapter revised from original article. Prasher, V.P., Farooq, A, Holder, R (2004). The Adaptive Behavior Dementia Questionnaire (ABDQ): Screening Questionnaire for dementia of Alzheimer's disease in adults with Down syndrome. *Research in Developmental Disabilities*, 25, 385–397. Printed with permission from Elsevier.

References

1. Heber, R (1961) A manual on terminology and classification in mental retardation (2nd edition). Am J Ment Defic, Monograph Supplement.
2. Gunzberg, HC (1977) Progress Assessment Chart of Social and Personal Development, SEFA Publications, Stratford-upon-Avon.
3. Nihira K, Foster R, Shellhas M et al. (1974) AAMD Adaptive Behaviour Scale, 1974 Revision, American Association on Mental Deficiency, Washington, DC.
4. Schupf N, Silverman WP, Sterling RC et al. (1989) Down syndrome, terminal illness and risk for dementia of the Alzheimer type. *Brain Dysfunction* 2: 181–188.

5. Brown FR III, Greer MK, Aylward EH et al. (1990) Intellectual and adaptive functioning in individuals with Down syndrome in relation to age and environmental placement. *Paediatrics* 85: 450–452.
6. Rasmussen DE and Sobsey D (1994) Age, adaptive behavior, and Alzheimer disease in Down syndrome: Cross-sectional and longitudinal analyses. *Am J Ment Retard* 99: 151–165.
7. Burt DB, Loveland KA, Chen Y-W et al. (1995) Aging in adults with Down syndrome: Report from a longitudinal study. *Am J Ment Retard* 100: 262–270.
8. Roeden JM and Zitman FG (1997) A longitudinal comparison of cognitive and adaptive changes in individuals with Down's syndrome and an intellectually disabled control group. *J Appl Res Intellect Disabil* 10: 289–302.
9. Prasher VP, Chung MC, and Haque MS (1998) Longitudinal changes in Adaptive Behaviour and Down syndrome: Interim findings from a longitudinal study. *Am J Ment Retard* 103: 40–46.
10. Nihira K, Foster R, Shellhaas M et al. (1969) Adaptive Behavior Scales. American Association of Mental Deficiency, Washington, DC.
11. Isett RD and Spreat S (1979) Test and retest and interratrer reliability of the AAMD adaptive behavior scale. *Am J Ment Defic* 84: 93–95.
12. Fogelman CJ (ed) (1975) AAMD Adaptive Behaviour Scale Manual. American Association on Mental Deficiency, Washington, DC.
13. Miniszek NA (1983) Development of Alzheimer's disease in Down's syndrome individuals. *Am J Ment Defic* 87: 377–385.
14. Collacott RA (1992) The effect of age and residential placement on adaptive behaviour of adults with Down's syndrome. *Br J Psychiatry* 161: 675–679.
15. Prasher VP and Chung MC (1996) Causes of age-related decline in adaptive behaviour in adults with Down syndrome; Differential diagnoses of dementia. *Am J Ment Retard* 101: 175–183.
16. Collacott RA (1993) Epilepsy, dementia and adaptive behaviour in Down's syndrome. *J Intellect Disabil Res* 37: 153–160.
17. Prasher V (1998) Adaptive behavior. In: Dementia, Aging, and Intellectual Disabilities, Janicki MP and Dalton AJ (Eds.). Taylor & Francis, Philadelphia, PA, pp. 157–178.
18. World Health Organisation (1992) The Tenth Revision of the International Classification of Diseases and Related Health Problems (ICD-10). WHO, Geneva.
19. Roth M, Huppert FA, Tym E et al. (1988) CAMDEX. The Cambridge Examination for Mental Disorders of the Elderly. Cambridge University Press, Cambridge.
20. World Health Organisation (1994) ICD-10 Symptom Checklist for Mental Disorders. Version 1.1. WHO, Geneva.
21. Aylward EH, Burt DB, Thorpe LU et al. (1997) Diagnosis of dementia in individuals with intellectual disability. *J Intellect Disabil Res* 41: 152–164.
22. Prasher VP (1999) Adaptive behavior. In: Dementia, Aging and Intellectual Disabilities: A Handbook, Janicki MP and Dalton AJ (Eds.). Taylor & Francis, Philadelphia, PA, pp. 157–182.
23. Zigman WB, Schupf N, Silverman WP et al. (1989) Changes in adaptive functioning of adults with developmental disabilities, Aust N Z J Develop Disabil 15: 277–287.
24. Evenhuis HM, Kengen MMF, and Eurling HAL (1990) Dementia Questionnaire for Mentally Retarded Persons. Hooge Burch, Zwammerdam, the Netherlands.
25. Prasher VP (1997) Dementia Questionnaire for Persons with Mental Retardation (DMR). Modified Criteria for Adults with Down syndrome. *J Appl Res Intellect Disabil* 10: 54–60.
26. Deb S and Braganza J (1999) Comparison of rating scales for the diagnosis of dementia in adults with Down's syndrome. *J Intellect Disabil Res* 43: 400–407.
27. Prasher VP, Huxley A, and Haque MS (2002) A 24-week, double-blind, placebo-controlled trial of donepezil in patients with Down syndrome and Alzheimer's disease—Pilot study. *Int J Geriatr Psychiatry* 17: 270–278.
28. Gedye A (1995) Manual for the Dementia Scale for Down Syndrome. Gedye Research and Consulting, Vancouver.
29. Burt DB and Aylward EH (2000) Test battery for the diagnosis of dementia in individuals with intellectual disability. *J Intellect Disabil Res* 44: 175–180.

Chapter 11
Strengths of Previous Work and Future Challenges

D.B. Burt

The dementia tests and scales described in previous chapters are an impressive representation of work conducted to improve dementia diagnosis in adults with intellectual disability (ID). In this chapter, the strengths of work represented in this book and anticipate future challenges are discussed. The discussion of strengths is not intended to be exhaustive. Instead, the following highlights and related future challenges will be considered: breadth of functional areas assessed within and across instruments, modified administration and scoring techniques, identification of dementia onset, monitoring of dementia progression, differential diagnosis, and scale evaluation methods. Additional general challenges faced by clinicians and researchers involved in dementia assessment include longitudinal research methods, multidisciplinary expertise, and funding.

Strengths of Previous Work

Breadth of Functional Areas Assessed

Other than tests designed specifically to assess one area of functioning (e.g., Cued Recall Test; Chapter 9), most of the instruments were designed to assess and document declines in several areas of functioning as required by dementia diagnostic criteria.[1] The most comprehensive assessment schedule, the Cambridge Examination for Mental Disorders of Older People with Down's Syndrome and Others with Intellectual Disabilities (CAMDEX-DS; Chapter 7), involves informant-report of functioning in a number of areas (e.g., memory, mental functioning, everyday skills), interview of the adult with ID, direct assessment of seven areas of cognitive functioning (e.g., praxis, language, memory), standardized observations of the adult with ID, and physical examination (including laboratory investigations). The schedule was designed to collect all information needed for a clinician to make a diagnosis of dementia over repeated assessments. Similarly, the informant-report dementia scales, the Dementia Questionnaire for Persons with Intellectual Disabilities (DMR; Chapter 3) and the Dementia Scale for Down Syndrome

V.P. Prasher (ed.), *Neuropsychological Assessments of Dementia in Down Syndrome and Intellectual Disabilities*,
DOI: 10.1007/978-1-84800-249-4_11, © Springer Science+Business Media, LLC 2009

(DSDS; Chapter 4) involve requests for information about multiple areas of functioning (e.g., orientation, social skills, memory performance). Informant-report scales for adaptive behavior also assess functioning in several areas (e.g., independent functioning, language development, economic activity; Prasher; Zigman and colleagues). Regarding direct performance tests, as an overall measure of mental status the Test for Severe Impairment (TSI; Chapter 8) assesses several functional areas (e.g., language, memory, conceptual ability).

The inclusion of multiple functional areas makes a scale more useful for several reasons. First, the scale is more likely to include areas needed to document declines for dementia diagnosis. Second, items/tests usually differ in terms of task demands (e.g., verbal vs. nonverbal responses). Thus, some of them are more likely to be useful than others for assessing adults with differing sensory abilities, premorbid levels of functioning, and strengths/weaknesses profiles. If an individual does not have or loses understandable speech, for example, items/tests that require nonverbal responses can be administered and scored separately. Multifaceted batteries or tests also allow the Examiner to create profiles of functioning to determine premorbid strengths and weaknesses. Decline may also occur at different rates for different skills across individuals. Such differences in the area and rate of decline were observed on the TSI and the Adaptive Behavior Scale (Prasher, Zigman, and colleagues).

To benefit from breadth in an assessment instrument, however, the instrument must allow documentation of performance on subscales or tests that assess different `recorded and available for future comparisons. One summary or composite score for all abilities is less useful than a set of scores, because declines in one but not all areas can be masked by a summary score. If so, then the summary score would be less sensitive to the onset of dementia than individual subtest scores. It is most useful if the repeated scores are raw scores as well as standardized scores and that they are accompanied by actual descriptions of performance (e.g., dresses self-completely including tying and buttoning, remembers five words in correct sequence in a sentence). In longitudinal research, instruments often undergo revisions which change the items included and the way summary scores are computed (e.g., the Maladaptive Subscale of the Adaptive Behavior Scale). On retest one needs to be able to compare current to previous performance and the more detailed the information, the more useful it will be. In addition, if an adult moves, the assessment procedures could change and with behavioral descriptions one can better judge whether changes in functioning have occurred.

In addition to strengths in the breadth of functional areas in individual scales, their breadth as a group is a strength. Several examples of dementia scales, adaptive behavior scales (standard vs. shortened version), and cognitive scales were presented. Challenges for future work are whether the scales would provide improved diagnostic accuracy if combined into a battery or schedule such as the CAMDEX-DS.[2,3] It is unknown at this time what combinations of scales allow optimal diagnostic accuracy for which adults with IDs. It is highly possible that different tests or groups of tests will be needed for adults with different characte-ristics (e.g., sensory abilities, levels of intellectual functioning, speech skills).

Administration Techniques

Another strength of the tests and scales was the innovative way in which adminis-tration techniques were developed and used. Multiple sources of information were described. In addition, flexible administration rules were standardized so that they would be appropriate for adults with differing capabilities.

Source of Information

As has often been the case historically, informant-report scales of adaptive behav-ior, everyday functioning, and emotional functioning were described. Direct assess-ments were described for tests of memory and other cognitive functioning. Such a dichotomous splitting of source of information allows a group of tests to be admin-istered to adults functioning at many levels and with different abilities. As long as informant-report and direct testing of adults are used to assess mutually exclusive areas of functioning (i.e., adaptive, everyday, emotional vs. cognitive, memory) all of which are involved in dementia diagnostic criteria, both sources of information will be needed to accurately assess dementia (Holland and Ball). Advantages and disadvantages of the use of the two sources of information were discussed by Burt in Chapter 2. Challenges for the future involve assessment of the veracity of informant reports and examination of ways in which to improve such reports.[4,5]

With the exception of the CAMDEX-DS, the adults with ID were not asked to report on their own memory, cognitive, everyday, or emotional functioning, nor were direct observations of functioning made a part of the assessment. Clinicians and researchers may routinely make observations or interview adults with ID as part of their clinical or research procedures. Such observations, however, were not integrated into the standardized scales or procedures themselves. Direct observation of the adult with ID is a critical part of any dementia assessment, and the standardi-zation of the observation and interview procedures is a strength because it allows procedures to be replicated and evaluated across sites.

An additional strength of informant-report work was the use of multiple informants to allow a determination of inter-rater reliability and the examination of differences in perspective (Prasher; Jozsvai and colleagues). The DSDS, for example, recommends informants from two different settings. Interestingly, there is a difference across scales in terms of the specified amount of time for reliable informants to have known the adult with ID. The DSDS requires that informants know the adult for at least 2 years, whereas the CAMDEX-DS interview requires only 6 months of association with the adult being described. In practice, unless adults with ID have close contact with parents or other family members, it is difficult to find an informant knowledgeable about all aspects of the adult's functioning. The length of time required for an informant to observe and adequately report on functioning for a dementia assessment is an area for future research and discussion. Promising work is already being done to train infor-mants to improve the accuracy and reliability of their reports.[5]

An additional strength of several of the informant-report scales is that informants indicated whether current functioning represents a change from typical functioning (Adaptive Behavior Dementia Questionnaire, ABDQ; Chapter 10, DSDS, CAMDEX-DS). It is very important to determine whether current behavior represents a decline or change from typical behavior as required by dementia diagnostic criteria. Such requests for judgments about typical functioning, however, often require a certain amount of retrospective reporting on the part of informants. Retrospective reporting is subject to memory errors or bias. As behavioral changes become more remote, it is possible that errors in memory will become more pronounced (e.g., the parent or other informant could forget what their child could previously do, adjusting their expectations to changing performance). At an initial evaluation for dementia, previous assessment information is not always available or in a format to allow for evaluation of changes in performance. Thus, retrospective reporting is the option of choice. It is beneficial as in the CAMDEX-DS, therefore, to allow informants to report that they don't know whether behavior is typical or not. They should also be allowed to respond that a question is not applicable to the adult in question. Such choices in responses are important so that an informant is not forced to make a response that does not accurately describe an individual.

Flexibility of Instructions

Investigators developed multiple forms of their scales or built in modifications to their administration procedures to allow for administration across individuals with different capabilities (e.g., sensory impairments, language spoken). Adminis-tration flexibility increases the applicability of the scale across individuals. It also makes it more likely that a scale will remain useful to chart the progression of dementia once skills are lost (e.g., loss of speech or the loss of a pointing response). Dalton, for example, built flexibility into the administration procedures for his Dyspraxia Scale for Adults with Down Syndrome (Dalton; Chapter 5). Instructions allow different levels of prompts for adults with differing sensory abilities. In this way, the Examiner is able to differentiate declines due to dementia from those due to sensory loss. Similarly, Holland and Ball made modifications to a number of the direct assessment items on the CAMCOG portion of their schedule. Points were awarded on the basis of answers given with and without the Examiner's prompting. Regarding considerations for differences in language or cultural background, Dalton built flexibility into his Dyspraxia Scale for Adults with Down Syndrome that allows for international administration (i.e., changing the coins used). The DMR allows flexibility in administration, because it is commercially available in Dutch and English (with other translations made for research purposes). Similarly, the DSDS is commercially available in English and French and has been administered in several non-English speaking countries such as Japan, Holland, and France.

Scoring

Approaches to scoring were innovative. Dalton, for example, computed *z*-scores for his Dyspraxia Scale, so that performance on it could be compared to performance on other tests in his battery. Mulryan and colleagues computed and examined annual rate of change scores on the TSI. Such scores provide a benchmark against which to compare repeated performance on the test. An examination of profiles of cognitive performance is possible on the CAMDEX-DS because of the derived subscale scores. Profiles of adaptive and maladaptive performance can be examined on the Adaptive Behavior Scale as demonstrated by Zigman and colleagues. Such comparisons allow an examination of the natural history of dementia. Relative decline is examined to see whether specifiable functional areas show decline first.

Innovative scoring procedures also allow one to determine which tests are best for screening early signs of dementia vs. later confirmation of dementia (i.e., documentation that diagnostic criteria are met). On the ABDQ, for example, Prasher used weighted item scores when he discovered that some items were more or less predictive of dementia than others. Such a weighting technique makes scales more useful and can make them adaptable for adults with different capabilities (i.e., if different weights are assigned based on level or cause of ID, age, gender).

It is important to remember that standardized scores, such as *z*-scores, must be interpreted with caution when they are obtained at one administration. Differences in scores could represent premorbid intraindividual differences in strengths/weaknesses profiles. If an adult with DS at one time of testing, for example, has strong dyspraxia performance compared to memory or fine motor performance it does not necessarily mean that the adult has had declines in memory or fine motor performance. It could be that dyspraxia has always been a relative strength for the individual. It is important to remember that there can be large interindividual differences in strength/weakness profiles as a function of sensory abilities, speech, and cause of ID (DS or other conditions). Such premorbid differences must not be confused with documented declines related to dementia.

Several investigators (Devenny and Krinsky-McHale; Zigman and colleagues) evaluated the use of cutoff scores or formulas to differentiate adults with dementia from those without dementia at one time of assessment. This procedure eliminates the need to rely on retrospective reporting (cf., ABDQ, DSDS). As mentioned by the investigators, however, there is usually overlap in the scores of adults with and without dementia. Consequently, a certain number of false-positive and false-negative diagnoses occur (as with any technique). The formula derived by Zigman and colleagues has the advantage of taking intelligence quotient (IQ) (when healthy) into account when interpreting performance. Cutoff scores used by Devenny and Krinsky-McHale were said to apply for adults with IQ scores of at least 30. On the DMR a single assessment approach, using different cutoff criteria as a function of IQ, was originally adopted and abandoned (Evenhuis and colleagues). Challenges for future work, therefore, will be to determine the advantages and disadvantages of using scoring systems designed for diagnosis based on one assessment.

As mentioned by Devenny and Krinsky-McHale, cutoff scores and formulas based on a research sample could be different than those needed for adults who have never seen the instruments or scales before.

Interpretation of scores from a dementia assessment is often a challenge. The inclusion of DSM-IV and ICD-10 dementia diagnostic criteria in a checklist, such as in the CAMDEX-DS, aids in the diagnosis and differential diagnosis of dementia. Such a checklist reminds practitioners that it is feasible to apply diagnostic criteria. It also provides a framework for reporting results from one assessment to another (i.e., which diagnostic criteria were met at a given time) and for comparing results across research studies. The CAMDEX-DS also provides guidance on how to use the information gained through the assessment in making a judgment about dementia status. Such guidance is valuable, because it is sometimes unclear how to use test scores either singly or in combination with others when making a diagnosis of dementia, or in deciding that a further dementia assessment is indicated.

Identification of Dementia Onset

The DSDS was designed to allow the clinician/researcher to identify the date of early skill loss, thus identifying the onset of dementia (Jozsvai and colleagues). The ability of informants to retrospectively report on the onset of first dementia signs, which can be gradual and difficult to detect, however, is a matter for future investigation.

Comprehensive procedures with repeated assessments, such as those from the CAMDEX-DS are designed to maximize the chances of detecting possible preclinical stages of an impending dementia. Extensive batteries and independent clinical assessments such as those used by Devenny and Krinsky-McHale, also allow an examination of early signs of dementia, such as preclinical changes in memory functioning.

Identifying the onset of dementia is important for clinical and research purposes. Detection of early changes indicates that the adult would benefit from differential diagnostic procedures such as those built into both the CAMDEX-DS and DSDS. Early change also indicates that the adult needs more extensive follow-up and monitoring than individuals without such change. Clinically, treatments could be most effective in the earliest stages of dementia if detection of such early changes is possible. In addition, if declines are related to some treatable condition (e.g., hearing loss due to ear wax or allergy-related congestion), then earlier detection leads to earlier treatment minimizing disruptions in functioning. For research purposes, if investigators are examining biological substrates of dementia, it is often necessary to detect the onset of clinical signs. If a certain biological process is associated with dementia, changes in a biological marker should coincide with or precede the onset of dementia. Regarding detection and description of preclinical changes, a challenge for future work is to determine the usefulness of terms used to describe preclinical decline (e.g., mild cognitive impairment, frontal type dementia).

Monitoring the Progression of Dementia

The ability to monitor the progression of dementia is a strength of several scales. The DSDS, for example, allows one to record ten assessments on the same form. The interval between repeat assessments is determined by behavior reported at each assessment. If signs of decline are reported, the interval between assessments is reduced to 6 months. Diagnostic accuracy improved on the DSDS with repeated assessment, so it is a strength of the scale to be able to record repeat observations on one form. The DSDS also provides guidelines to identify stages of dementia based on the scores obtained at each assessment.

As mentioned previously, comprehensive schedules like the CAMDEX-DS and multiscale batteries (Devenny and Krinsky-McHale; Zigman and colleagues) allow one to detect declines in functioning and to determine when some but perhaps not all diagnostic criteria are met.[2,3,6] Such schedules allow one to describe the natural history of dementia across individuals to determine whether there is any universal pattern or invariant sequence of decline. The DMR also provides separate scores for cognitive vs. social functioning, and subscale scores in each area can be recorded. Thus, the Examiner can determine whether changes occur in both areas simultaneously or whether declines in one area precede the other. Holland and Ball suggest that changes in personality or behavior precede cognitive changes. Zigman and colleagues suggest that maladaptive changes precede changes in adaptive behavior and that within the adaptive behavior domain not all skills decline at the same rate. Devenny and Krinsky-McHale indicate that declines in Cued Recall Test (see Chapter 9) occur early. Mulryan and colleagues conclude that declines in delayed memory, writing ones name, and counting to 10 precede well-practiced motor tasks like shaking hands. Additional research is needed at multiple sites to determine whether there is an invariant progression of decline in adults with and without DS with dementia and whether stages will be identified such as those reported on the DSDS. As demonstrated by the work here, declines can only be detected in areas being assessed repeatedly. If an investigation in cognitive/memory change does not assess early personality or behavioral changes, for example, it is difficult to determine the actual sequence of decline.

Differential Diagnosis

The inclusion of techniques in a scale to aid in differential diagnosis is valuable. The techniques highlight the fact that conditions other than Alzheimer disease cause changes in functioning. It is the clinician/researcher's responsibility to consider all possible causes of any behavioral changes, and to provide treatment or to refer adults for treatment as appropriate. As with many of the procedures involved in a comprehensive dementia evaluation, attention to differential diagnosis may be standard practice for most clinicians/researchers. The inclusion of standardized procedures for their consideration, however, ensures that they will not be overlooked and allows others to replicate and evaluate them. Two assessment instruments contain techniques to aid in differential diagnosis. The DSDS includes questions to help in the identification of conditions such as hypothyroidism and depression. The CAMDEX-DS provides a structure to collect information on physical conditions, psychiatric disorders, and sensory impairments that can affect functioning in later life. Holland and Ball also provide case studies to illustrate that conditions such as hearing difficulties or depression affect functioning. The CAMDEX-DS also provides guidance for postdiagnosis intervention, highlighting the fact that the diagnosis of dementia is just the beginning of the clinical process.

Evaluation Methods

Impressive techniques were used to evaluate dementia tests and scales. Investigators, for example, used external criterion for dementia status that were independent of the scale being evaluated (Devenny and Krinsky-McHale, Holland and Ball, Prasher). Holland and Ball also used their direct assessment data to evaluate their interview schedule, and thus were able to avoid possible errors involved is using clinical judgment as the sole external criterion. Investigators also used extensive diagnostic procedures to determine that adults identified with dementia did not have other conditions that could account for declines (e.g., depression). When examining DAD specifically, investigators also ruled out other types of dementia. In addition, scales and dementia identification criteria were developed using one sample of adults, and then evaluated in completely independent samples (Prasher) or in samples of adults with new onset dementia (Devenny and Krinsky-McHale, Zigman and colleagues).

A number of techniques were used to make scales more efficient and accurate. Prasher, for example, discerned that some of the items on his scale were less useful than others, so he eliminated them (i.e., reports of toothbrushing skill). Devenny investigated ways to shorten the assessment process by evaluating the use of two vs. three trials of data. Holland and Ball eliminated items from the original CAMCOG that were less useful for the assessment of adults with ID (e.g., serial sevens). Dalton combined data on his Dyspraxia Scale from several sites, so that he could determine which items were most useful. He then shortened the scale to improve efficiency and ease of administration. Evenhuis compared the value of single vs. repeated administration of the DMR, and changed her recommendations regarding optimal testing schedule based on her findings. She also determined that her scale was most useful in the midrange of ID, because of floor and ceiling effects in adults in the profound and mild levels of functioning, respectively.

Scales have been used and evaluated at numerous sites (Adaptive Behavior Scale, DMR, DSDS, and TSI). Thus, evidence is accumulating as to their validity and reliability. The DSDS, for example, has been used in a number of research studies, with evidence suggesting that it is most useful for adults similar to the normative sample who are functioning in the severe or profound range of ID.

A future challenge is whether the scale needs modification to increase its sensitivity across a wider range of capabilities. The DMR has also been evaluated in a number of studies, with some inconsistency regarding the usefulness of single vs. repeated administration. Such multisite evaluation is the type of valuable research that is needed to determine the usefulness of existing and newly developed dementia scales.

Instruments were identified as being most useful as either screening or diagnostic tools. The CAMDEX-DS and the DSDS were designed and evaluated for the diagnosis of dementia. In contrast, the Dyspraxia Scale for Adults with Down Syndrome, the DMR and the ADBQ were described as screening instruments that could be used to detect early signs of dementia. The Cued Recall Test detects preclinical or early declines in memory (Devenny and Krinsky-McHale) suggesting that it would also be useful in a battery to screen for dementia. Assessment of maladaptive behavior (Zigman and colleagues) could also be useful in a dementia screening battery. Future research is needed to determine the combination of screening and diagnostic tools that will lead to early, efficient, and accurate diagnosis of dementia in adults with ID.

Future Challenges and Directions

Several challenges in future work for clinicians and researchers were mentioned in the discussion of the strengths of previous work. Three additional challenges related to the longitudinal methods needed to examine dementia assessment procedures are now discussed.

Longitudinal Research

There are several challenges inherent in the longitudinal assessment required to evaluate dementia scales (i.e., repeated assessment over time). The first challenge is to integrate collection of useful baseline data into assessments that are already being conducted for adults with ID (e.g., transition to workplace assessment in the United States). Logistic issues also arise, such as storing information/data for long periods of time in a format that is useful. Another logistic issue is the loss of investigators, who lose funding or become older themselves and retire from clinical or research work. One issue illustrated by several of the investigators (e.g., Evenhuis and colleagues; Dalton; Prasher; Zigman and colleagues) is change in scoring techniques or scale modification over time. A clinician/researcher could collect and store information about adults in one format. They could, for example, store data indicating whether adults meet cutoff scores for dementia on the DMR on the basis of one assessment, total scores on the full Dyspraxia Scale for Adults with Down Syndrome, and total scores on the adaptive behavior scale. If the clinician/ researcher then wanted to use the newly modified scoring criteria, they would have to change their scoring procedures (i.e., use only change scores on the DMR, use the shortened dyspraxia or adaptive behavior scale scores; use the maladaptive behavior scale with improved reliability). Such modifications are only possible if the clinician or researcher has access to previously collected raw data. Data or clinical information must be stored in a form as close to that which was collected as possible to allow for maximum usefulness across time.

Interdisciplinary Expertise

Longitudinal, cutting-edge research on dementia assessment requires expertise across a number of disciplines. Given that dementia diagnosis is a clinical judgment (Holland and Ball; Prasher; Jozsvai and colleagues), it is imperative that someone on the clinical/research team has actual experience with the challenges of diagnosing dementia in adults with ID. Using clinical judgment improves with time and experience. Developing and evaluating dementia assessment scales requires further expertise. Unfortunately, clinicians and researchers with an interest and expertise in the diagnosis of psychiatric disorders in adults with ID are rare. Training programs for their education are also rare. The type of research needed, involving repeated assessment of the same procedures, is not the type of innovative, creative process that easily attracts and holds the attention of researchers. Communicating extensively with other researchers and integrating methods across sites is not a commonly taught skill. From a research standpoint, a relatively small number of participants with dementia of the Alzheimer type are identified after years of costly research. Thus, researchers who are sometimes required to compete with each other for funds and publication space are going to need to collaborate across sites to make true progress. It is difficult to attract clinicians and researchers to the field of dementia assessment in adults with ID in the first place, and then retaining them is another challenge.

When conducting evaluations of instruments or diagnostic methods, members of the evaluation team need to be up to date on research and statistical methods needed to examine longitudinal data. There are a number of issues to be considered and research is ongoing to better illustrate what are typical or atypical patterns of performance over time. Test–retest effects, for example, must be considered[7] as well as the effects of attrition due to death or survival due to above average health.[8] In conducting analyses to examine the sensitivity, specificity, and predictive validity of instruments or techniques, it is important to remember that how one defines dementia has considerable effects on these measures. For example, if adults with diagnoses of possible dementia are included in a group with dementia, the results could be very different than if such adults were excluded all together or considered to be in the not demented group. It is sometimes helpful to be flexible in terms of analyses, by conducting them several different ways to see if diagnostic grouping has significant impact on conclusions drawn. A dementia diagnosis involves judgment, and it is best to remember that one is evaluating groupings that are almost certain to contain some erroneous assignment of adults (i.e., false-positive or false-negatives). A team member who is cognizant of changes related to aging vs. those related to dementia is a valuable asset to help in making decisions about group assignment. Finally, an area for future research is the examination of associations between test performance and any biomarkers that aid in the diagnosis of dementia (Dalton; Zigman and colleagues). Once again, members of the research team or consultants to the team would need the expertise required to perform such research.

Funding

Interested researchers and clinicians find it difficult to acquire funding for their assessment work. As mentioned, longitudinal research designed to examine instruments to assess dementia is costly, and consistency is currently more important than creativity. A number of scales and instruments have been developed and a logical next step is a large collaborative evaluation of them. Clinicians who are also researchers are in an ideal position to collect and examine data if funding is available (e.g., Prasher, Holland, and Ball). To obtain such funding, in the United States, however, it could require a grassroots call for funding like that launched regarding autism diagnostic issues in the last several years.

Dalton demonstrated the usefulness of incorporating scale evaluation in clinical trials. Such work could have greater funding potential than assessment evaluation research, but the researcher must have the interest and tenacity required to make scale assessment a subsidiary goal of the research. Researchers have the responsibility to make the greatest use of data collected. The need to share data further illustrates the need to store data in formats that others can use, both for scale development and evaluation purposes (e.g., Dalton). Such sharing requires clinicians/researchers to take a leadership role in fostering scale development and evaluation. The ability to provide such leadership requires energy, tenacity, experience, and expertise such as that demonstrated by the authors in this book.

Conclusions

In conclusion, the clinicians and researchers whose work is represented in this volume have made outstanding progress toward improving dementia diagnostic accuracy for adults with ID. There are considerable future challenges for additional strides to be made. At present, competitive work is being done with researchers making progress at various sites. Cross-site collaboration occurs occasionally. Perhaps it is not realistic to expect collaboration across national boundaries, when such collaboration does not exist for dementia assessment in the general population. The relatively small size of the population of adults with ID and dementia, existing disparities in the quality of health care, and the need for active advocacy for needed research indicate that collaboration in the population with ID will be required. Leaders in the area need to convene international workgroups to generate goals for dementia research in the next decade and beyond, and to identify mechanisms to reach such goals.

References

1. Aylward EH, Burt DB, Thorpe LU et al. (1997) Diagnosis of dementia in individuals with intellectual disability. *J Intellect Disabil Res* 41: 152–164.
2. Burt DB, Primeaux-Hart S, Loveland KA et al. (2005) Comparing dementia diagnostic methods used with people with intellectual disabilities. *J Policy Pract Intellect Disabil* 2: 94–115.
3. Burt DB, Primeaux-Hart S, Loveland KA et al. (2005) Tests and medical conditions associated with dementia diagnosis. *J Policy Pract Intellect Disabil* 2: 47–56.
4. Burt DB, Primeaux-Hart S, Phillips NB et al. (1999) Assessment of orientation: Relationship between informant report and direct measures. *Ment Retard* 37: 364–370.
5. Ball SL, Holland AJ, Huppert FA et al. (2004) The modified CAMDEX informant interview is a valid and reliable tool for use in the diagnosis of dementia in adults with Down's syndrome. *J Intellect Disabil Res* 48: 611–620.
6. Holland AJ, Hon J, Huppert FA et al. (2000) Incidence and course of dementia in people with Down's syndrome: Findings from a population-based study. *J Intellect Disabil Res* 44: 138–146.
7. Thorvaldsson V, Hofer SM, Berg S et al. (2006). Effects of repeated testing in a longitudinal age-homogeneous study of cognitive aging. *J Gerontol: Psychol Sci* 61B: P348–P354.
8. Hawkins BA, Eklund SJ, James DR et al. (2003) Adaptive behavior and cognitive function of adults with Down syndrome: Modeling change with age. *Ment Retard* 41: 7–28.

Appendix 1
Questions on Clinical Usefulness of Scales, Tests, and Techniques

(A) Practical issues

- How much time is required for completion of the scale or technique (e.g., assessment battery) at each assessment?
- Is the scale completed in one assessment or does it require repeated assessments over time? If the scale requires repeated assessments, is clinically useful information obtained at each individual assessment?
- What cost is involved? Is any technology involved (e.g,, computers with special programs)?
- What level of expertise is required to administer and interpret results from the test? How much clinical judgment is required to determine whether an adult has dementia (declines in functioning) or not? If more judgment is required, more expertise and experience is needed and one could expect greater differences across raters.
- What source of information is being used, the adult with ID or an informant?

(B) Purpose

- Is a particular scale or technique designed to aid in formulating a diagnosis of dementia (e.g., dementia scales), or is the technique designed to determine whether one of many diagnostic criteria have been met (e.g., memory tests, adaptive behavior scales)?
- Does the scale clearly indicate performance that would be indicative of dementia vs. performance that would not?
- Does the scale provide a dichotomous classification (dementia vs. no dementia) or does it provide an indication of possible dementia?
- Is the technique designed to detect all types of dementia or just progressive dementia like that associated with Alzheimer's disease?
- Has the scale been evaluated to see if it is a good indicator of early signs of dementia, as in a screening test? Or is the scale better suited as a confirmation that dementia is present?
- If the scale indicates stages of dementia, to what extent were such stages validated (i.e., all adults pass through the same stages, only adults with certain types of dementia pass through them, only adults with certain etiologies of ID or premorbid levels of functioning pass through them)?

- Is there a series of questions or techniques designed for purposes of differential diagnosis (e.g., to identify untreated thyroid disease, depression[1])?
- If the test is an assessment of one area of functioning, has it been evaluated as part of a larger batter to see if sensitivity, specificity, or predictive value are improved.[4]
- If the scale or technique involves the combination of several skills into one test (e.g., a test with memory and other cognitive components) are scores for each component skill available?
- Have statistical vs. clinically significant differences in functioning been diffe-rentiated?[1]
- Can the test be applied in different countries with appropriate translation, or are the items culture specific? Has the technique been evaluated across sites, languages, and cultures?
- If the technique is an adaptation of one used in the general population, has it been modified appropriately so that it is applicable to adults with ID?

References

1. Gedye A (1985) Dementia Scale for Down Syndrome. Manual. Gedye Research and Consulting, Vancouver, BC.
2. Burt DB, Primeaux-Hart S, Loveland KA et al. (2005) Comparing dementia diagnostic meth-ods used with people with intellectual disabilities. *J Policy Pract Intellect Disabil* 2: 94–115.
3. Burt DB, Primeaux-Hart S, Loveland KA et al. (2005) Tests and medical conditions associ-ated with dementia diagnosis. *J Policy Pract Intellect Disabil* 2: 47–56.
4. Silverman W, Schupf N, Zigman W et al. (2004) Dementia in adults with mental retardation: Assessment at a single point in time. *Am J Mental Retard* 109: 111–125.
5. Devenny DA, Zimmerli EJ, Kittle P et al. (2002) Cued recall in early-stage dementia in adults with Down's syndrome. *J Intellect Disabil Res* 46: 472–483.

---

[1] Perhaps in a research setting, it has been determined that a decline on a memory test of two items is outside the range expected with normal aging. Would all adults with such a decline have dementia? With such a small indication of decline, any adult who does not recall two items when healthy could not meaningfully be assessed on the test. For this reason, tests with a large range of performance across all adults with ID are often recommended. With memory tests, for example, repeated presentation of test stimuli usually results in higher performance and a larger range of scores.[2,3,5] This makes the test more useful for dementia assessment. The use of memory cues has also been found to improve performance.[5]

Appendix 2

DMR

Category	1	2	3	4	5	6	7	8
1. Understands what you want to make clear to him/her (by means of speaking, writing or gesticulation): 0 = normally yes / 1 = sometimes / 2 = normally no								
2. Remembers where he/she put away something just a minute ago (no longer than half an hour ago): 0 = normally yes / 1 = sometimes / 2 = normally no								
3. Remembers an impressive event that took place during the last weeks (tells about it or recognition is apparent from behaviour when it is spoken about): 0 = normally yes / 1 = sometimes / 2 = normally no								
4. Knows which month it is (e.g. March in the first week of April is permitted): 0 = yes / 1 = sometimes / 2 = no								
5. Remembers family members or friends whom he/she has not seen for a long time or who are deceased: 0 = yes / 1 = sometimes / 2 = no								
Total page 2								

"Special abbreviated version of the Dementia Questionnaire for People with Intellectual Disabilities, produced after written permission dated 6-07-2006 by the publishers Harcourt Assessment B.V., Amsterdam, The Netherlands. info@harcourt.nl.

Appendix 3
Scoring Sheet for the Dyspraxia Scale for Adults with Down Syndrome

DYSPRAXIA SCALE FOR ADULTS WITH DOWN SYNDROME
SCORING SHEET

NAME _____

LOCATION _____

SEX _____

AGE _____

DOB _____

EXAMINER _____

DATE EXAM _____

Part 1: Psychomotor Skills

While standing

No.	Item Score	4	3	2	1	0
1	Walking					
2	Standing					
3	Look up					
4	Bend your head					
5	Bow from waist					
6	Clap hands					
7	Lift one arm					
8	Lift other arm					
9	Turn head one side					
10	Turn head other side					
11	Lift one leg					
12	Lift other leg					
13	Sitting					

While seated

No.	Item Score	4	3	2	1	0
14	Draw a circle					
15	Draw straight line					
16	Clip two sheets					
17	Cut paper sheet					
18	Three coins (one hand)					
19	Coins (other hand)					
20	Put on cap/take off					
Subtotals						
Part 1 Total						

Part 2: Apraxia

No.	Item Score	4	3	2	1	0
21	Make a fist					
22	Salute					
23	Wave good-bye					
24	Scratch your head					
25	Snap your fingers					
26	Close your eyes					
27	Sniff a flower					
28	Use a comb					
29	Use a toothbrush					
30	Use a spoon					
31	Use a hammer					
32	Use a key					
33	Open a jar					
34	Close a jar					
35	Put on right glove					
36	Put on left glove					
37	Unlock padlock					
38	Lock padlock					
39	Fold sheet of paper					
40	Fold sheet again					
Subtotal						
Part 2 Total						

Part 3: Body Parts/Coin Task

No.	Item Score	4	0
41	Point to your ear		
42	Point to your nose		
43	Point to your eye		
44	Point to your chest		
45	Point to your neck		
46	Point to your chin		
47	Point to your thumb		
48	Point to your ring finger		
49	Point to your index finger		
50	Point to your little finger		
51	Point to your middle finger		
52	Point to your right ear		
53	Point to your right shoulder		
54	Point to your left knee		
55	Point to your left ankle		
56	Point to your right wrist		
57	Point to your left elbow		
58	Point to your right cheek		
59	Give me a penny		
60	Give me a nickel		
61	Give me a quarter		
62	Give me a dime		
Part 3 Total			

Appendix 4

PART ONE
DOMAIN I.
Independent Functioning

A. Eating

ITEM 1 **Use of Table Utensils**
(Circle highest level)

Uses table knife for cutting or spreading 6
Feeds self neatly with spoon and fork
(or appropriate alternate utensil, e.g., chopsticks) 5
Feeds self causing considerable spilling with spoon and
fork (or appropriate alternate utensil, e.g., chopsticks) 4
Feeds self with spoon—neatly 3
Feeds self with spoon— considerable spilling 2
Feeds self with fingers 1
Does not feed self or must be fed 0

ITEM 2 **Eating in Public**
(Circle highest level)

Orders complete meals in restaurants 3
Orders simple meals like hamburgers or hot dogs 2
Orders single items, e.g., soft drinks, ice cream, donuts, etc.
at soda fountain or canteen 1
Does not order in public eating places 0

ITEM 3 **Drinking**
(Circle highest level)

Drinks without spilling, holding glass in one hand 3
Drinks from cup or glass unassisted—neatly 2
Drinks from cup or glass unassisted—considerable spilling 1
Does not drink from cup or glass unassisted 0

ITEM 4 **Table Manners**
(Circle all answers)

If these items do not apply to the individual, e.g., because
he or she is bedfast and/or has liquid food only, place a
check in the blank and mark "Yes" for all statements. ____

	Yes	No
Throws food	0	1
Swallows food without chewing	0	1
Chews food with mouth open	0	1
Drops food on table or floor	0	1
Does not use napkin	0	1
Talks with mouth full	0	1
Takes food off others' plates	0	1
Eats too fast or too slow	0	1
Plays in food with fingers	0	1

B. Toilet Use

ITEM 5 **Toilet Training**
(Circle highest level)

Never has toilet accidents 4
Has toilet accidents only at night 3
Occasionally has toilet accidents during the day 2
Frequently has toilet accidents during the day 1
Is not toilet trained at all 0

ITEM 6 **Self-Care at Toilet**
(Circle all answers)

	Yes	No
Lowers pants at the toilet without help	1	0
Sits on toilet seat without help	1	0
Uses toilet tissue appropriately	1	0
Flushes toilet after use	1	0
Puts on clothes without help	1	0
Washes hands without help	1	0

C. Cleanliness

ITEM 7 **Washing Hands and Face**
(Circle all answers)

	Yes	No
Washes hands and face with soap and water without prompting	1	0
Washes hands with soap	1	0
Washes face with soap	1	0
Washes hands and face with water	1	0
Dries hands and face	1	0

ITEM 8 **Bathing**
(Circle highest level)

Prepares and completes bathing unaided 6
Washes and dries self completely
without prompting or helping 5
Washes and dries self reasonably well with prompting 4
Washes and dries self with help 3
Attempts to soap and wash self 2
Cooperates when being washed and dried by others 1
Makes no attempt to wash or dry self 0

ITEM 9 **Personal Hygiene**
(Circle all answers)

If these items do not apply to the individual,
e.g., because he or she is completely dependent on
others, place a check in the blank and mark "Yes"
for all statements. ____

	Yes	No
Has strong underarm odor	0	1
Does not change underwear regularly by self	0	1
Skin is often dirty if not assisted	0	1
Does not keep nails clean by self	0	1

ITEM 10 **Toothbrushing**
(Circle highest level)

Cleans dentures appropriately 5
Applies toothpaste and brushes teeth
with up and down motion 5
Applies toothpaste and brushes teeth with
sideways motion 4
Brushes teeth without help, but cannot apply toothpaste 3
Brushes teeth with supervision 2
Cooperates in having teeth brushed 1
Makes no attempt to brush teeth 0
Does not clean dentures 0

D. Appearance

ITEM 11 **Posture**
(Circle all answers)

If these items do not apply to the individual, e.g.,
because he or she is bedfast or non-ambulatory, place
a check in the blank and mark "Yes" for all statements. ____

	Yes	No
Mouth hangs open	0	1
Head hangs down	0	1
Stomach sticks out because of posture	0	1
Shoulders slumped forward and back bent	0	1
Walks with toes out or toes in	0	1
Walks with feet far apart	0	1
Shuffles, drags, or stamps feet when walking	0	1
Walks on tiptoe	0	1

195

Appendix 5

MEMORY AND ORIENTATION

Memory

42	a)	Does he/she have difficulty remembering recent events e.g. when he/she last saw you or what happened the day before?	Yes 1	➜	b)	Is this a deterioration?	Yes ➜	Slight deterioration 1
			No 0				No 0	Great deterioration 2
			DK 8				DK 8	
			N/A 9				N/A 9	
		Examples of change:						

43	a)	Does he/she often have difficulty remembering where he/she has left things?	Yes 1	➜	b)	Is this a deterioration?	Yes ➜	Slight deterioration 1
			No 0				No 0	Great deterioration 2
			DK 8				DK 8	
			N/A 9				N/A 9	
		Examples of change:						

44	a)	Does he/she have difficulty remembering what has been said and repeat the same question over and over?	Yes 1	➜	b)	Is this a deterioration?	Yes ➜	Slight deterioration 1
			No 0				No 0	Great deterioration 2
			DK 8				DK 8	
			N/A 9				N/A 9	
		Examples of change:						

45	a)	Does he/she have difficulty in remembering short lists of items, e.g. shopping?	Yes 1	➜	b)	Is this a deterioration?	Yes ➜	Slight deterioration 1
			No 0				No 0	Great deterioration 2
			DK 8				DK 8	
			N/A 9				N/A 9	
		Examples of change:						

46	a)	Does he/she have difficulty remembering significant events from his/her past?	Yes 1	➜	b)	Is this a deterioration?	Yes ➜	Slight deterioration 1
			No 0				No 0	Great deterioration 2
			DK 8				DK 8	
			N/A 9				N/A 9	
		Examples of change:						

We Acknowledge Ball et al. (2006). Page 16. CAMDEX-DS. Cambridge University Press

Appendix 6

Case Study 1—John

Background/best level of functioning

- John is 54 years old and lives in a group home with eight other residents.
- Has attended a day center for the last 10 years and used to help in the kitchen at lunchtimes.
- He is active socially, attending church, a social club, and going to the pub on a weekly basis.
- He has a group of friends and a best friend.
- He likes to watch Startrek on the TV and enjoys coloring.
- He never learned to read and has only ever been able to copy his name.
- At his best level of functioning, he was able to prepare meals and carry out housework independently, and took care of grooming, dressing, and personal hygiene without assistance.

Changes reported by carer

Everyday skills

- He used to help in the kitchen at his day center but is unable to do this anymore because he gets muddled.
- He now needs much more prompting to perform everyday household chores and needs reminding how to do things.
- He used to be able to cook independently but only helps out now and can only prepare simple snacks independently, e.g., toast.
- He needs prompting at each stage to make a cup of tea. This is a big change.
- He used to go shopping in a group but now requires one-to-one supervision as he needs prompting as to what to buy, and will pick up items that he does not need.
- These changes have occurred gradually over the last **6 months.**

Other cognitive skills

- He finds it much more difficult to concentrate on things. He needs prompting halfway through activities.
- His thinking processes seem to have slowed down and his thinking seems muddled.
- He has word finding difficulties and often muddles words up that he used to know, using the wrong word.
- He has difficulty following instructions, particularly if too many instructions are given at once, and needs prompting at each stage.
- He has difficulty completing complex sequences of actions, e.g., household chores, cooking, dressing.
- He has difficulty planning ahead. He used to pack his bag for day center the night before but no longer thinks ahead and bag is packed for him.

- He has difficulty making decisions, e.g., what he would like to eat for dinner. He just says "don't know" or "don't mind" when given a choice.
- These changes have occurred gradually over the last **12 months**.

Personality/behavior

- He shows inappropriate behavior in public, e.g., shaking hands with strangers. This is a change from usual behavior, since he used to be quite shy.
- He shows less concern for others, e.g., not noticing when other residents are unwell.
- Has become more stubborn, awkward, and uncooperative, particularly when reminded to do things he used to be able to do.
- He has started to repeat the same phrase over and over again.
- Gradual changes over last **12 months**.

Memory

- He has much greater difficulty remembering recent events, e.g., if asked what he did yesterday, he wouldn't remember that he went swimming. This is a major change.
- He forgets what has been said and repeats the same question over and over again. This has become much more noticeable recently.
- He has great difficulty in remembering short lists. He used to remember a short list of items to buy at the shop but can no longer do so.
- He often loses his glasses or other personal items. This is a slight change from previous behavior.
- He has become confused about what day it is. He used to remember which day he went to his social club but doesn't remember anymore.
- Sometimes he thinks it is morning in the middle of the night (for the last 3—4 months).
- He is aware of his memory problem and often frustrated by it.
- These changes have happened gradually over the last **12 months**, escalating more rapidly over last **6 months**.

Self-care

- He has difficulty dressing, gets things in the wrong sequence and often forget items. He now requires a moderate degree of assistance but used to be completely independent.
- He now wets and soils himself. Always used to get to toilet on time.
- He needs much more prompting when combing hair and shaving. Moderate assistance required now but used to be independent.

older people, cleaning at a pub, and a work placement at a furniture project. He had also received training in essential skills at college.

- He has never been able to read. He is able to write his name and copy.
- He has a very active social life, attending a drama group, a social club, and going to the pub at least once a week. He has many hobbies, listening to music, snooker, darts, dominos, gardening, and DIY. He has many friends without learning disabilities.
- At his best level of functioning he has been able to shop independently for small purchases, perform light housework tasks, prepare snacks, and heat up meals. He is independent in grooming, dressing, and personal hygiene.

Changes reported by carer

Everyday skills

- He requires more prompting to carry out his activities at work and on placements. He has less confidence in his abilities and has become very sensitive about errors he makes.
- He requests more supervision/prompting to perform everyday household chores, which he used to do independently, and in his hobbies—gardening and DIY.
- He needs to be washed, as can now only wash hands and face. He used to be independent in the bath.
- Gradual changes over **6 months**.

Mental health

- He talks more slowly than he used to.
- No other signs of depression or other mental illness.

Physical health

- No sensory difficulties.
- No other physical health problems.
- Doesn't take any medication.

Case Study 2—Michael

Background/best level of functioning

- Peter is 52 years old and lives in supported housing with one housemate.
- He attended special school until the age of 15 and since then has held a number of jobs including working in a shoe factory, making tea and washing up at a residential home for

- These changes have occurred gradually over the last **18 months**.
- He is able to shop independently for small purchases, dial a few well-known numbers on the telephone, prepare snacks, and heat things up in the microwave. There is no decline in these abilities.

Memory

- There has been no change in his ability to remember recent events.
- He asks the same question again but only when he doesn't understand the answer!
- Has never been able to remember lists.

Other cognitive skills

- He finds it much more difficult to concentrate on things and gets easily distracted. He needs much more prompting for things he used to do independently.
- His thinking appears to be slower and more muddled than it used to be.

- He has difficulty making decisions and changes his mind a lot. He did not used to do this.
- He is less confident about making decisions/solving problems by himself—he used to do gardening, and DIY by himself but now asks for more supervision.
- These changes have occurred gradually over the last **18 months**.

Personality/behavior

- He has become much more sensitive, e.g., if he does something wrong he has tearful moments—this has been noticed at his place of work (on a furniture project).
- He has become more changeable in mood.
- He has become more irritable and angry, particularly toward his housemate.
- He shows less concern for others' feelings.
- He has become more stubborn. Won't be hurried into doing things.
- He no longer enjoys colouring or cross-stitch (which he now says is a woman's activity!).
- He repeats the same phrase over again "Where you been?" (6 months)
- Gradual changes over last **18 months**.

Self-care

- He has no difficulty in dressing, but requires prompting to change his clothes.
- There has been no change in grooming or other self-care skills

Mental health

- Sometime he cries for no apparent reason. This is a change.
- He finds it more difficult to concentrate that usual for him.
- Gradual change over **18 months**.
- NB: He is currently on antidepressant medication.
- He complains unjustifiably of being picked on, but this has always been the case.
- Has always talked to himself and seen visions of animals such as rats. He does not believe these are real.

Physical health

- He has a hearing problem, but this is corrected with a hearing aid.
- He has no other physical health problems and doesn't take any medication.

Case Study 3—Mary

Background/best level of functioning

- Mary is 51 years old and lives in a residential home with five other residents (has been there for last 3 years).
- She did not attend school and entered institutional care at age 10. She is severely learning disabled and has only ever had very limited speech. She has never been able to read and write. She has attended college for a sensory music and movement group in the past.
- She is not involved in many activities outside the home. She occasionally goes shopping—in a wheelchair. She has always been "in her own little world." However, she enjoys singing and has a best friend who she lives with.
- At her best level of functioning she was able to use the toilet independently and walk independently. She was not able to perform any household tasks, and has been dependent on others for major assistance with dressing, bathing, and grooming.

Changes reported by carer

Everyday skills

- She used to love singing and knew the words to songs. Does not know the words anymore and sings less often.
- She no longer attends the sensory, music, and movement course due to difficulties attending. She used to go on the bus but now has problems with mobility and takes no more than a few steps, supported by another person.
- Change has occurred gradually over the last **12 months**.
- She has never been able to perform any household tasks.

Memory

- Her memory has always been poor. Also, it is very difficult to judge how much she remembers, due to limited speech. She has never used people's names.
- However, she has much greater difficulty knowing where she is/interpreting surroundings—she used to recognize when she was in the bathroom, but now she does not.
- She has much greater difficulty finding her way round the home.
- She forgets what time of day it is and gets up during the night.
- These changes have been gradual over the last **6 months**.

Other cognitive skills

- Her thinking seems to have slowed down though it has always been muddled.
- She talks much less than she used to.
- These changes have occurred gradually over the last **12 months**.

Personality/behavior

- She has become much quieter and more withdrawn.
- She has also become much more stubborn, e.g., refuses to go in the bath.
- She has lost interest in things going on around her and does not show as much emotion as she used to.
- Gradual changes over last **12 months**.

Self-care

- She used to be able to feed herself independently, but now needs to be fed.
- She now wets herself quite often (more than once a week). This did not used to happen.

- These changes have occurred gradually over the last **6 months**.

Mental health

- She shows a lack of interest in things in general.
- She has lost her appetite and lost weight in the last 6 months.
- She is less sociable than she used to be.

- She sleeps a lot by day.
- Gradual change over **12 months**.
- No other signs of depression or other mental illness.

Physical health

- She has cataracts.
- She has suffered from seizures for the last 2 years.
- She is taking antiepileptic medication.

Appendix 7
Test For Severe Impairment

NAME_____   ID Number_____
DATE_____   AGE _____

Write down all responses verbatim that are different from those on the sheet. If *S* does not hear a question or is distracted, you may repeat the question up to three times in order to engage their attention.

Motor Performance

Comb
"Show me how you would use this comb"
Hand **S** comb
Correctly demonstrates combing   1___
Pen and Top
"Can you put the top on the pen?"
Remove the top from the pen in full view of **S**
Hand the pen and top to **S**
Correctly puts top on pen (not on bottom of pen)   1___
Pen and Paper
"Write you name"
Hand **S** pen (without the top) and place paper on
table in front of **S**
Writes name correctly (first or last name legible)   1___

TOTAL 3   ___

Language—Comprehension

"Point to your ear"
Correctly points to ear   1___
"Close you eyes"
Correctly closes eyes   1___
Pens—Red, Blue, Green
"Show me the red pen,… the green pen"
Place the three pens on the table spread out so that they have some space between them
Correctly points to red pen   1___
Correctly points to green pen   1___

Total 4   ___

Language—Production

"What is this called"
Point to your nose
Correctly names nose   1___
Pens—Red, Green
"What colour is this pen"
One at a time hold up a (red, green) pen in front of *S*
Correctly names red   1___
Correctly names green   1___
Key
"What is this called"
Show *S* the key
Correctly names key   ___

Total 4   ___

Memory—Immediate

One large paperclip
"Watch carefully"
Place clip in your hand so *S* can see
Hold hands out to *S*
With hands open
"Which hand is the clip in?"

Correctly points to clip 1   ___
With hands closed
"Which hand is the clip in?"
Correctly point to hand with clip 1   ___
Move hands behind back
"Watch carefully. Which hand/side is the clip in/on?"
Correctly points to hand with clip   1___

Total 3   ___

General Knowledge

"How many ears do I have?"
Correctly states two   1___
"Count my fingers and thumbs"
Place hands in front of *S* with fingers pointing up,
palms toward *S*. Credit given even if no 1 to 1
correspondence between fingers and numbers.
If *S* only gives final answer, ask, "Can you count
to 10 starting at 1?"
Correctly counts to 10   1___
"How many weeks are there in a year?"
Correctly states 52   1___
"I'm going to sing a song. If you know the words,
I want you to sing along with me." Softly sing "Happy Birthday."
Sings most of the words   1___

Total 4   ___

Conceptualization

Two large paperclips, one pen
"Which one of these is different form the other two"
Spread objects on the table.
Correctly points to pen or states pen   1___
Two red pens, one green pen
"Put this next to the pen that is the same colour"
Place 1 red and 1 green pen spread out on the table
Hand *S* the other red pen
Correctly places the red pen next to the other red pen   1___
One large paperclip

Place hands out in front of **S**
Alternate the clip between the opens hands 4 times
"Watch me move the paperclip
Which hand will I put the clip in next?"   1___
After **S** responds, place clip in correct hand
If **S** is incorrect say "I'd put the clip in this hand"
Then say, "Which hand will I put it in next?"
Correctly points to correct hand   1___

Total 4   ___

Memory—Delayed

Thread, key, paperclip
"Which one of these haven't we done something with
while you were here with me?"
Place objects spread out on table
Correctly points to thread   1___

Total 1   ___

Motor Performance

"Thank you for spending time with me"
    Extend hand to shake hands
    Correctly shakes hands   1___
Total 1   ___

Tsi Total Score = 24   ___

Appendix 8
The Adaptive Behavior Dementia Questionnaire (ABDQ)

Name:_____ Date of Birth:_____

	Question	Answer			
1	Are they able to dress themselves?	Better than normal	Same as normal	Worse than normal	Much worse than normal
2	Can they use their hands to do things?	Better than normal	Same as normal	Worse than normal	Much worse than normal
3	Is their ability to buy things?	Better than normal	Same as normal	Worse than normal	Much worse than normal
4	Are they able to have a conversation?	Better than normal	Same as normal	Worse than normal	Much worse than normal
5	Is their awareness of time?	Better than normal	Same as normal	Worse than normal	Much worse than normal
6	Do they help to prepare food?	More than normal	Same as normal	Less than normal	Much less than normal
7	Do they help to clear the table?	More than normal	Same as normal	Less than normal	Much less than normal
8	Are they able to perform simple jobs?	Better than normal	Same as normal	Worse than normal	Much worse than normal
9	Can they initiate things/ activities?	More than normal	Same as normal	Less than normal	Much less than normal
10	Is their ability to persist in doing things?	Better than normal	Same as normal	Worse than normal	Much worse than normal
11	Can they take care of their belongings?	Better than normal	Same as normal	Worse than normal	Much worse than normal
12	Do they cooperate with requests?	More than normal	Same as normal	Less than normal	Much less than normal
13	Do they carry out simple commands?	Better than normal	Same as normal	Worse than normal	Much worse than normal
14	Do they participate in group activities?	More than normal	Same as normal	Less than normal	Much less than normal
15	Is their ability to do things independently?	Better than normal	Same as normal	Worse than normal	Much worse than normal

Index

Printed in the United States